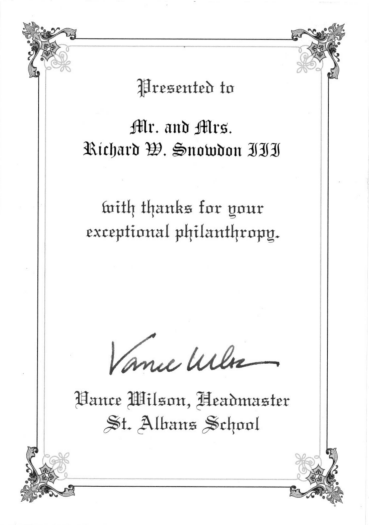

Presented to

Mr. and Mrs.
Richard W. Snowdon III

with thanks for your
exceptional philanthropy.

Vance Wilson, Headmaster
St. Albans School

ROOM FOR IMPROVEMENT

Contents

Preface

People occasionally ask me why on earth I keep on doing what strikes them as a painful exercise at what strikes them as an advanced age. There's no single answer. One thing I'm sure of is that it's not masochism.

I recently had a conversation with a philosophical trainer in a gym. He said that most people have some kind of addiction. Some use "exogenous stimulants"—booze or drugs. Some people use "endogenous stimulants"—chemicals produced by their own bodies. Some of them are hooked on getting angry, falling in love, or taking risks. He thought I was lucky to be hooked on endorphins, the secretions released by the human body after a half hour or so of cardiovascular exercise. Endorphins are also released by people making love and pregnant women.

The philosophical trainer and I agreed that neither health nor vanity would be enough to keep us going. But I don't think endorphins, as pleasant a feeling of well-being as they provide, would be enough, either. There's something else. I'm not sure what that something else is. In the course of going over older essays on various sports and exercises and my forty-two years of logbooks, I think that there is more than one something. There is health (both physical and mental). There is vanity—

wanting both to look good and to be skillful, perhaps even feel graceful. Endorphins, check. Playfulness—sometimes it's just fun to feel like an otter. Adventure. Adventure includes being ready to say yes if someone says, "You want to climb Mount Katahdin?" Or "You want to canoe down the Delaware River?" Or "You want to run a marathon?"

And there's getting into the woods. A student of mine once asked me, "What is it with you and nature?"

I answered more or less like this: "I wouldn't write if I didn't read a lot. I also wouldn't write if I didn't get out in the physical world in my own body, sometimes as a 'sojourner in nature,' as Thoreau puts it, but sometimes pushing hard enough to see and feel the earth's surface differently. Thoreau did that, too. He hiked the Maine woods, climbed Mount Katahdin, walked great lengths of Cape Cod, went down the Merrimack River in a small boat. He wasn't looking for near-death trips, and neither am I. 'The bear went over the mountain . . .' There's a lot to see along the way."

Adventure also includes competition. Competition against others, against oneself, against challenging conditions. You have to read your opponent; you have to read a river.

I also found an additional dimension of friendship in team sports, a mostly wordless confidence and comradeship. This is particularly true of rowing in every size racing boat—eights, fours, quads, pairs, and doubles. In an eight and a four I've often felt deep affection for a good coxswain. I imagine it's something like what a racehorse feels for a good jockey—though, as I note later, animal-to-human communication is a tricky business.

Being useful in practical ways seems to come up last—but not least. Double-digging a vegetable bed, pruning trees, sawing firewood (it would be faster with a chain saw, but I love my old long crosscut saw with wicked large teeth). I got in shape for a long canoe trip by digging out the silt from my flooded cabin—two hours a day for ten days. I was surprised that my pulse rate was as high as it gets when I am jogging, and surprised at how cheerful I was. Endorphins? Or just the satisfaction of taking care of things?

Redemption. There's redemption of a bad day at the writing desk. Okay, that was five hours of nothing—let's blow it off by running five miles.

There's also longer-term redemption. The subject of this book is exercise, from middle age into old age, but there are half-buried memories of feeling puny and humiliated. In his plump middle age, Cyril Connolly wrote, "Inside every fat man there is a thin man wildly signaling to be let out." A reverse of that notion is that inside every grown man, no matter how apparently at ease, there is a cringing little boy hoping to be kept in.

When I was thirteen I went to a boys' canoe camp in Ontario. The base camp was on an island in Lake Temagami, at that time, 1952, still mostly uninhabited. We canoed and portaged over a good bit of Ontario, sometimes traveling thirty miles in a day. We didn't see any people or houses. I loved the lakes and rivers. I loved seeing moose, ducks, black bears. We wore few clothes. We were in seven canoes—eleven boys, a counselor, an assistant counselor, and a guide (Stan Meilleur, who admitted he was the best guide in Ontario, maybe in all of Canada. I thought he was). All but two of us boys were fifteen or fourteen. Two of us, Schuyler van Kimball and I, were thirteen. We were the only ones without pubic hair, the ones still with little-boy tinklers. I was nicknamed Buddha for my fat tummy and chest. I also stuttered.

One evening after pitching the tents we all went swimming.

As usual, we went in bare. As we got out, one of the fifteen-year-olds said, "Who's got the smallest dick—van Kimball or Casey? Anybody got a ruler?" Another fifteen-year-old said, "Wouldn't work. But we could use the links on the little chain Ward's got his Virgin Mary medal on."

I dove back in and swam out twenty yards. I stayed there until it was dark.

At the end of that summer I went to a Swiss boarding school. All the classes were in French, except, of course, for English. The month after starting to learn French, I was called on in history class to give a summary of the Trojan War. *"Les G-g-grecs étaient fâchés parce que P-p-paris a volé Heh-heh . . . Hélène."*

The school took three days off for All Saints'. We were put into teams of four for a competition that was part scavenger hunt, part orienteering. The clues were left all over Switzerland—one at the Berne Zoo, another at the Basel post office, then in smaller villages, and finally in the Alps. The clues were in French, German, Italian (the three official languages), and Latin and English. There were a number of English, Canadian, and American boys among the hundred and twenty students. Reale, an Italian, was our team leader. As at Camp Keewaydin, I was the youngest and shortest, no longer plump but still so squat I was almost square.

During the last leg of the trip we had to climb a hill. It seemed endless. It began to snow. My shoes, unlike Reale's boots, didn't have nubbly soles. I was wet from head to toe, and lagging behind. The higher we went, the deeper the snow. It was dark when we reached the rendezvous, a large chalet. Our team came in last. After supper we sat on the floor. The headmaster told us we were going to move on another few kilometers to a large barn near a Swiss Army camp. The headmaster added, "If there is anyone who thinks he can't keep up, my wife has room in her car. By road it is longer, so we will arrive at the same time. Raise your hand if you wish to ride in the car."

I was in the front row, beside a small Indian boy. He raised his hand. I raised mine. We were the only two.

The other boys started off. Sat, short for Satrahalisinji, and I were consoled by Madame Johannot. Sat had never seen snow. I had no excuse.

The next day I kept to myself. The headmaster, like all Swiss men, was in the Army Reserve, a major. He arranged that we be allowed to fire rifles under the supervision of the Swiss noncommissioned officers. They had set up balloons on the far side of a gorge. Any volunteers? A few of the older boys stepped forward. Everyone else seemed shy. Were they afraid of guns? I raised my hand. The headmaster raised his eyebrows. He finally nodded. I thought I could redeem myself. I'd shot .22 rifles since I was seven. I had a sharpshooter model from the NRA.

The older boys shot first. They couldn't hit the broad side of a barn door. The rifles were bolt-action, took a clip of eight rounds and one in the chamber. The Swiss noncoms had been putting in single rounds. I pointed to the clip. The noncom looked at the headmaster. He looked dubious. I said, "*Je sais f-f-faire ça.*"

"*Voyons alors. Vas-y, Casey.*" He pronounced it *Kah-zay*.

One balloon. Work the bolt. Two. Work the bolt. Three . . . Nine shots, nine balloons.

What did I expect? That my contemptible weakness would be erased? That someone would clap me on the back? There was only uneasiness. Nothing was erased. Instead something was added on. I was a show-off. And something else. Some confirmation of the European suspicion that all those American movies weren't fantasy. America *was* Al Capone and Jesse James. If armed, even a squat little twerp might have a vicious streak.

In the winter the school moved from the shore of Lake Geneva to the mountains. During the Christmas break those boys who lived very far away stayed in the school's chalets. I spent hours ice-skating by myself on the enormous outdoor rink. I watched the hockey players. The school had a number of teams, one of which was made up of faculty members and three Canadian boys. It played in the Swiss national league. Not the NHL—Switzerland is small—but still . . . The star of the team was Monsieur Rupik. He'd left Czechoslovakia after the Communists took over. He'd played on the Czech Olympic hockey team. He was a rarity in that he'd also been on the Czech Olympic rowing team. He coached cross-country running in the fall (his hero, not surprisingly, was Emil Zátopek), hockey in the winter, and rowing in the spring. He was admired, even idolized. I knew him only from afar, as I wasn't a likely candidate for cross-country.

One day Monsieur Rupik skated over to me. The second-string goalie was missing. Would I put on the goalie pads?

Monsieur Rupik suited me up, gave me the right-hand blocker glove, the left-hand catching glove (that was familiar—like a first baseman's mitt). He showed me how to hold the goalie stick, and then the scrimmage was on. I stopped a few shots just by standing there. Then a shot came in slightly to the left. I caught it and flipped it behind the cage. Monsieur Rupik gave me a pat on the shoulder. After the scrimmage he asked me to stay for a bit. He and a Czech friend of his named Bruno spent an hour shooting pucks at me. They taught me how to play goalie—that day and every day of the Christmas break. Monsieur Rupik called me *opicak*, Czech for hedgehog—I was small and had a bristly crew cut. He also told me to practice skating on my own—lots of short bursts and stops.

When school started in January I played goal for the under-fourteen team. When we went to the schoolboy championships in Zermatt, I also played on the under-sixteen team, whose goalie was sick. We lost in both finals, but my teammates said encouraging things, which by now I could understand.

Just before the Easter vacation I went skiing with two friends. We were walking back through the village with our skis on our shoulders. In a shop window I saw a reflection. Three boys—there was Paolo Serra, and Antony Velie, but who was the third? *I* was at the far end, taller than Serra or Velie. No longer pug-nosed, chubby-cheeked, and squat. I'd had a growth spurt, a usual thing for someone turning fourteen. Like Pinocchio, I'd wished and wished to become a real boy. I thought it was something I owed to Monsieur Rupik.

In the spring Monsieur Rupik asked me to row. The fourteen-and-under four were Winthrop, Casey, Hadley, and Watson, four Americans. An advantage of being an American born in 1939 or 1940 was having been safe and well fed. (These days Italian kids are taller than their parents, tower over their grandparents. The new generation is called *i vitaminizatti.*)

I took to rowing. I would have taken to anything for Monsieur Rupik. I can still hear his Czech-accented French. *"Longue dans l'eau!"* Or, if our strokes weren't exactly synchronized, *"C'est une mitrailleuse!"* (A machine gun.) If we still didn't get it right, *"C'est un bordel!"* (A whorehouse—not as shocking in French as it is in English, just a tangier way of saying it's a mess.)

What would unredeemed fourteen-year-old boys do without a Monsieur Rupik?

ROOM FOR IMPROVEMENT

I Got Fat in Law School

I got fat again in law school. I lost endurance and agility. The low point was a pickup softball game. I played third base, fielded a ground ball but wildly overthrew to first base. Then I ran for a pop foul and fell headlong in the dirt, a spectacle that got laughs from the business-school team.

I'd been a high-school athlete, football, soccer (at that time a winter sport), and track and field (100, 220, hurdles, shot put, javelin)—small school, small track team. We multitasked. I plumped up spring of sophomore year in college, went mildly nuts, got kicked out. I got back in shape during basic training at Fort Knox from the usual marching and bayonet drill, plus playing flag football on the Company C, Ninth Regiment, third training division team. The team captain was Second Lieutenant Hal Greer, then just out of college, soon to play guard for the Philadelphia 76ers. Hal Greer was a superb athlete. When he turned the corner on an end run, he had an extra gear. Running interference for him, I'd sense him behind me, and then he'd be gone. He also took our flag-football games totally seriously. One of my jobs was to get between him and the referee when he was outraged at a bad call. He said, "Don't let me get thrown out of the game, Private. I authorize you to take hold of me."

The high point of my season was when Lieutenant Greer threw me a pass in the end zone. I dove for it, caught it, and tucked it in as I fell. Lieutenant Greer yelled, "Casey! You're not a dud!" Still sweet a half century later.

The team's name was The Night Fighters. Lieutenant Greer may have thought this up. It certainly wasn't me or the only other white boy on the team, a fireplug lineman who'd played for Massillon High School in Ohio. It was flag football, but there was all-out blocking, and nipping the flag from the ball carrier's web belt often involved tackling. We won the post championship, mainly because Lieutenant Greer was our company's executive officer and pushed the team members during calisthenics and bayonet drill. He kept his eye on us in the field, encouraging us to *run* rather than do the easy Army double time when we were asked to deliver a message to the first sergeant or company commander. We learned to volunteer. Lieutenant Greer had an edge, and he willed us to have an edge.

Back to college, on to law school. A decline from catching a touchdown pass to sprawling out of reach of a pop foul.

After law school, I went to work for a congressman. I kept a strange schedule. Day of work at the office, bar-exam prep course in the evening, at night jogging to a track and running a mile, then two. Then I took to the Chesapeake and Ohio Canal towpath on weekends. Nowadays there's a crowd of joggers and bicyclists. Back then a lot of people out for a stroll stared or made jokes ranging from corny ("Hey there—you training for a race or racing for a train?") to rude ("Aren't you kinda hefty to be running in this heat?").

After a while I got leaner and fast enough not to hear more than a word or two—either that or I began to get "runner's high," the onset of endorphins (though I didn't know the word then), and was encased in the rhythm of what I was doing.

The Social Life of the
Long-Distance Runner

I wrote "The Social Life of the Long-Distance Runner" more than forty years ago. The title is a play on "The Loneliness of the Long Distance Runner," a grim story and a grim movie, one that only film buffs and older people remember. When I reread this piece I found it in several places very young—both strainingly lyrical and wiseass—but it reminded me that in the late sixties there were few joggers, and those few attracted wiseass remarks. The essay was the first piece in a national magazine about what was to become a widespread pastime. On the canal towpath in Washington, D.C., there are now more joggers than walkers, and no one gives them a second glance. There are places in the world where the sight of bare legs and arms is still shocking. An old student of mine got run in by the moral police in Saudi Arabia for jogging in Bermuda shorts. There are lots of joggers in Rome but mainly in parks. Once when I was jogging back to my apartment through Testaccio, an older woman, in black from head to toe, called out to me, *"Coprati, coprati, giovanotto!"* (Cover yourself, cover yourself, young man!) I was fifty-one, pleased to be called *giovanotto.* She may have been offended by bare skin, or she may have been expressing the national cold phobia. Two generalizations about Italians are true: they love children and fear cold drafts. Old women and men often told me to put more clothes on my two small daughters. They said, *"Prenderanno un raffredore"* (They'll catch cold) and then lovingly patted their cheeks. *"Che carina!"* (How darling!)

I f you walk through any of the parks in Washington during the warmer months, you are likely to see apparently masochistic young men running by you, their faces sweaty, flushed, and tortured, their mouths gasping noisily for air, their motley outfits flapping wetly against their legs and backs as they heave along. Why do they do it? For future glory on the playing fields, you may imagine, for sport, for manly beauty, for Spartan well-being. But not—unless something is awfully wrong—for pleasure.

I thought so as well. From my soccer-playing days I remembered running laps, wind sprints, and other devices of tedium and torture, designed, it seemed at the time, to weed out the unenthusiastic. It is true that friends of mine, usually longer-legged and somewhat reedy, had described attaining a certain pleasurable trance while running long distances, but I had put them in the same category as people who sat through two consecutive showings of *Last Year at Marienbad.*

However, on a day a spring or so ago that I was spending in the field with my Army Reserve unit, two sergeants appeared to give a lecture on physical fitness. They said that the Vietcong could travel, trotting stealthily along in their tennis shoes, forty miles a night. The sergeants invited us to run along with them for just a few miles. They set a brisk pace, littering their trail with us until they shed the last body before the three-mile mark. They still had enough breath to retrace their steps and insult each of us individually. I will not say it was cause and effect, but that summer I took up distance running through the parks near my house. First downhill.

Battery Kemble Park runs from Foxhall Road to MacArthur Boulevard for a distance of about a mile and a quarter, most of it parallel to Chain Bridge Road. The only disadvantage to running down through the park is that you have to climb back up. At that time, *running* back up seemed out of the question.

I got into the habit of doing a mile and a fraction a day—faster and faster but always downhill. There had been scarcely any pain. After a week I was emerging from my jaunts not breathing any harder than when I first kissed a girl good night.

I soon realized that this wasn't really a workout—I was just skimming the cream. At that time I was employed by a congressman by day, studying for the bar exams at night and feeling very virtuous about my exercise between the two. But two things happened. First, the football players from American University joined me in Battery Kemble for their preseason conditioning. They ran down *and* back in football shoes. Second, I was reading A. J. Liebling on boxing, and he informed me that one of the lesser boxers held down a full-time job, did gym work for three hours, *and* ran five miles in Central Park. He did his five miles in forty-five minutes. It was clear that my manager wasn't bringing me along fast enough. Between boxers, football players, and the Vietcong, the world was still too fast for me. So I started running back up. I was glad when the bar exams came so I could stop. And yet there was . . .

yes . . . a new pleasure in scrambling up the last hill. Part of it was that I could feel my thigh muscles spurting right out of my otherwise abundant flesh. But there was also a less spartan and more luminous joy.

It was shortly after this that I hit upon the notion of trying a level run, and the place I selected was the towpath along the old Chesapeake and Ohio Canal.

My sweat suit was still in the wash, so I put on old khakis over a pair of shorts. I treated myself to new wool socks that gleamed like golden cream in contrast to my sneakers, which were skillfully camouflaged dirt-brown and held together with gray adhesive tape. I drove down to Chain Bridge. I climbed down the stairs to the towpath and hid my khakis under them. My plan was simple. I would run the 3¼ miles to Key Bridge and then trot up 34th Street, ringing doorbells of friends until I found one who would drive me back to my car.

I breathed deeply, looked at my watch, and sprang nimbly down the towpath.

The first spectators emerged from the woods and onto the towpath in front of me after only a quarter of a mile. Leading them was a very pretty girl of about twenty-four. Holding each of her hands were two small children, and trailing behind them were a dozen others, both male and female. Third or fourth grade, I guessed. As I came within earshot, their teacher released her hands and herded them all to one side. "Oooh, children," she said, spreading her bare arms like a traffic-safety director, "look at that. A track star!"

"Yeah," one of the little boys sneered. "Here he comes to save us in his Keds." The schoolteacher giggled.

Even my bar-exam-numbed brain realized that I was the butt. As I went by, the little girls shrieked and grabbed their skirts. Their teacher twitched her mouth at them and said,

"Shh." Slowing down, I said, "Madam, you have a lovely family." More little shrieks from the girls and cackles from the boys. One little boy, however, shouted fiercely at my back, "She's not *old* enough to be our mother!" And, with just a catch of a pause, he added, "Stupid!"

"Tommy!" the teacher said with just the right mixture of shock and affection.

After another quarter mile I looked back. They were wandering toward Chain Bridge. I could see no one in front of me, only a raw stretch of empty towpath.

It's a little depressing being able to see where you'll be after ten or twenty minutes of fairly strenuous exercise, but there was a compensation in being by the canal. There is a hypnotic effect in running by flat, still water. It is deeply peaceful, especially in the light of a late-summer afternoon. There isn't a stretch of anything else in the whole city that is so level, so long, and so straight. The air hanging softly over it was peaceful, too, trembling only occasionally like a billowed net held in place by spars of sunlight that stemmed from between the trees on the southwest side of the path. I was the only graceless movement.

I ran for a while with my eyes turned to the left over the canal. I had been practicing a little autohypnosis. It helps to repeat to yourself seven times or so, "I am light, I am barely touching the ground, I am floating swiftly forward." It takes your mind off the ploddingness of it all. I succeeded so well that I was in a sort of trance. I began to think that if I suddenly swerved to the left I would run right across the water. It wasn't that it looked solid. On the contrary, everything was light. Beams, spots, and layers of light. The canal was not deep; it was nothing but a surface—blankets of light, some dull and some splattered with pieces of sun, all laid jaggedly side by side for miles. The treetops projected against the sky seemed no more real than the slightly darker ones lying across the dusty golden water.

And I was nothing but a patch of bright movement. Without looking down, I still caught glimpses of my clean wool socks chasing each other over the dirt path. They looked like those pieces of reflection you sometimes see on the wall of a shuttered room that overlooks a busy street in summertime. It may be the outside mirror on a car or the front window of a bus that throws the bright spots up through the vents of the shutter, but the spots have an existence all their own as they skitter across the wall; grow long, slinking around the corner; and skim across pictures or curtains or onto the ceiling.

That was the way I was beginning to feel about my feet and the darker canal. Skim right across. No trouble at all. *Why not try?* said the same voice that tells me to jump off high buildings.

I was saved from total immersion and its consequent lingering tropical diseases by a sudden gap in the towpath. I had to swerve to get onto a wooden footbridge that crosses a small ravine. And at the other end of the footbridge there was a body.

It was a man, facedown, his hands tucked under his belly. I finally managed to derail myself about fifteen yards beyond him. I turned around, still jogging, and approached.

"Hello!" I said in a loud voice. Nothing happened. I stood still for a moment. *They'll blame it on you,* said my small voice, probably irritated at not having landed me in the canal. I rolled the man over by his shoulder.

The man's face was bright pink on the top half and white stubble on the bottom. He didn't move. I was feeling for his pulse when one eye opened.

"Awragh, a short nap," he said clearly, although all that seemed to move was the one eye.

"Sorry," I said.

"*Per*fectly all right," he said, opening his other eye. "Ah, my friend," he continued, "you look old enough to wind a chronometer . . ."

"What?"

". . . but all in good fellowship, let me tell you as one who has seen . . ." He stopped and closed both eyes. I stood up. ". . . As one who has seen," he said, "the best and the worst. Don't sign the ticket." He opened one eye.

"What?" I said again.

"Never sign the ticket. All the little redheads. All the little blondes. All of them. All of them, my friend." He sighed deeply. "Never sign the ticket. Squeeze them. Fondle them. Caress them. Kiss them. Even beat the hell out of them. But never . . ."

"Sign the ticket," I said, anxious to be on my way.

"That's right!" he said, opening both eyes with delight at my aptness. He started in again.

"I've got to go," I said.

"*Per*fectly all right," he said, "*per*fectly all right. Unless by chance you have the kindness to offer me"—he closed his eyes—"a free sample of the coin of the realm."

"I'm awfully sorry," I said.

"That's perfectly all right, my young friend," he said, his eyes fluttering open once more. "*You* are a connoisseur of the protocols; *I* am a connoisseur of the vicissitudes." As he whistled the last word his eyes opened all the way to the deep red moats that surrounded them.

I was a little sorry to leave when he was just getting warmed up, so I turned and waved back after I had trotted off a few steps.

"Very good," he said loudly. "Keep running. Keep running—that's what keeps the world spinning."

As I ran along, the spires of Georgetown University appeared high on my left. The spires used to remind me of Cardinal Richelieu, because as a child I used to think that he lived there. Nowadays I can never see them without also thinking of the monsignors who do, and who, strolling slowly to and fro in their soutanes, wish that he really did.

I was clopping along at a good pace, so caught up with my vision of government under the red cloak that I was startled to see two mules advancing toward me along the gentle curve of the towpath. Beside them was a muleteer, and behind them a large barge with a peaked striped awning.

I swerved onto the grassy fringe of the path far away from the mules. I thought mules might bite.

On board there was a cocktail party. Forward, a full-bellied man in a colorless summer suit leaned across the railing and pantomimed offering me a drink. The girl beside him laughed excessively, clutching her gin and tonic to her, her curled fingers against her breastbone, the top of the glass right under her chin.

They were all there—all the little redheads, all the little blondes, and all the little brunettes—standing slimly under the awning in linen sheaths, bright green and pink and cream. One blonde in the port-stern quarter had her arm twined around a pole like bunting. She smiled a beautiful white smile at me and held out a canapé of black caviar. She made an underhand tossing motion and raised her eyebrows invitingly. I frowned seriously. She laughed from beneath her shiny hair, which spouted in opposing question marks from a part in the middle.

The women were visibly superior to the men. The men were scarcely more than shadows, except for a brilliant tie or two. But even the women didn't come close to those lovely Renoir women along a Renoir river. These elbows were too pointed. And you couldn't have painted *these* hips and bottoms with a sturdy brushstroke—it would have been an exaggeration. You could have done each slender body with a pastel shaving. And the men with a sponge dipped in rinse water.

Having laughed, my blond friend made a pretty pout just as we reached our perigee. Another second and we would never see each other again, but I felt I had a message for her. "Never sign the ticket" was perseverating in my brain. I growled at her, however, "The future belongs to the fit."

Another peal of laughter. Then she stuck her tongue out.

Just before I reached the bridge I saw a fisherman on the opposite bank. He was tall, dressed in Army fatigue pants and an Eisenhower jacket. When I was thirteen I spent almost a whole week fishing in the canal. I thought I should convey the results to him.

"Hello!" I shouted. "There aren't any fish in there. You'd better go over to the river."

"Heh, heh," he said, holding up a string of four fat fish.

"They must have stocked it," I said, not quite so loudly.

"Heh, heh," he said again.

I jogged up the steps to street level. My eyes were suddenly assailed by a battery of headlights sweeping off M Street onto the bridge. Along the street there were still some old-fashioned globe streetlamps on their ten-foot Corinthian pillars of ornamental iron painted municipal gray, but mostly there were the new-fashioned arc lights—the kind that turn red-lipstick purple. They perch on the curb like praying mantises and hover their mandibles fifteen feet over the roadway, cutting off the sky. Very insectlike and ominous.

I caught the traffic light on the run and crossed over to trot up the other side of M Street in the gutter so I would not have to weave through pedestrians. I got a few strange looks, but not as many as I did when I began to ring doorbells on 34th Street, jogging in place on the front stoops while I listened to the distant unanswered ringing.

I condemned the whole lot of my friends as useless gadabouts. Not one was in. I finally found myself marking time in front of 1606 34th Street, which is about six blocks up the hill. I felt a little silly. Also betrayed. Even if you don't phone ahead, you expect people to know you're coming. All the more so if you've run the whole way. I sighed and started back. I nurtured the illusion of a second wind, like a man lighting a cigarette with one match on a windy day. I trundled down the hill to Key Bridge. The brightness of the intersection still gave me a shock. I skipped across, breathing through my nose. I thought that would filter the exhaust fumes better. The real shock, however, came when I finished threading myself down the narrow stairs. It was dark down there. I could practically lean on the blackness.

After a while it was extraordinarily quiet. All I could hear was the crunch of my shoes on the dirt. That helped me settle into a rhythm, and since I couldn't see my feet land, I achieved a floating sensation without going through the usual liturgy. I began to imagine that the darkness wasn't resisting me anymore but that, having accepted me, it gave way before me and even squeezed from behind, making a favorable current. I was happy to graduate from mystic biology to mystic physics; I imagined that I was being helped by a pre-Einsteinian ether drift. It got so good that I even began thinking of the towpath as one of those old-fashioned vacuum tubes that used to suck up sales slips to the money room and whoosh back a plush capsule filled with your change.

While all this mind drift was going on, the moon climbed over the tops of the trees on the far bank. I saw that I was halfway to Chain Bridge when the light hit an old landmark—the skiff that once was used as a ferry across the canal. I also suddenly felt like walking. I slowed down a little and peered ahead, trying to see the retaining wall and the footbridge. There was a rustling under the bank just ahead of me, and then a peeping and scurrying. Three long rats ran across the path in front of me and disappeared into the woods. I spurted ahead. Even when I slowed down again I still would prance skittishly back to the middle of the path if I drifted to one side or the other. I began to think of all sorts of venomous things—rabid dogs lying in wait, red-bellied swamp spiders, copperheads. It wasn't the DT's, but it kept me on my toes. After a period of five minutes or so, I settled down again. I settled down so completely that I nearly stopped. I began to inquire whether it was possible for there to be a third wind. Glancing down at my feet, I saw my white socks passing mysteriously over the ground like determined ghosts. Encouraged, I thought, *Yes—any minute now.* There was an ache in my right shoulder every time I breathed.

I checked my feet, which were still stepping out confidently, still ghostly, and I felt something like a third wind. "I could go on forever," I said out loud for my benefit. But I was running with both slower and shorter strides—and very heavily—when I saw, some distance ahead, a light moving sideways. It was a car crossing the bridge. I postponed my final sprint for a dozen strides while I tried to figure exactly how far it was. Then, a little ashamed of myself for being lazy, I stretched my stride and began, as they say, my kick. *Aha!* I thought. *There's lots left.* I ran so that I could hear the wind in my ears, but the bridge and I seemed to be getting no closer. I ran harder, my mouth open and my eyes watering. *I could go on forever,* I thought, this time in despair. Then the bridge jumped to a reasonable distance, and after a few more seconds I thudded past the bottom of the stairs. *"Nike,"* I said, and breasted the tape.

I turned around and shuffled back. I found my long pants, unrolled them, and started to put them on. I lifted one leg and fell down. Instead of sensibly staying on the ground, I kept getting up, lifting one leg and falling down. Finally I sat down on the steps and got the pants on. I pulled myself up the stairs and along the bridge railing. I tried walking without holding on and weaved out to the curb and back to the railing. I sat down on the sidewalk for a minute, remembering to check for the car keys. I had just found them in my back pocket—the one that buttoned—when a car door opened in front of me. The man who got out was dressed in navy blue.

"Hello there," I said.

The policeman in front of me bent down and sniffed. He called back, "He don't smell drunk." He said to me, "Breathe out."

I started to get up. He lowered his hand on my shoulder with a friendly pat. "Don't get up—just breathe, Charlie. You don't look steady on your feet."

I breathed. He sniffed.

"I try to brush after every meal," I said.

He held my arms and used his flashlight to check them for needle marks.

"Better call in," he said to his friend. The driver blew into the microphone. "Pweh, pweh," he said. "This is car oh-seven, car oh-seven, at point . . ." He leaned across the seat and asked us, "Where are we?"

"This is Chain Bridge," I said.

"Point A-five," my friend said.

"Why don't you just say Chain Bridge?" I asked. He didn't say anything. You would think that they'd like to talk to someone besides each other.

"Pweh, pweh, A-five. We've got an unidentified suspicious male putting his pants on. White, medium build, medium complexion, medium height . . ."

"I'm a shade over six feet," I said.

"Settle down, Charlie."

". . . in khaki pants and a T-shirt . . ."

"It's a Pancho Segura tennis shirt," I said. "He is famous for his two-handed backhand."

My friend smiled, and I smiled back. "Shut up," he said. I realized he was grinning at the thought of shutting me up.

"Do you have any complaints?" the driver asked into the microphone.

We sat around awhile until the radio announcer said, "Brakh, brakh, oh-seven, oh-seven, negative."

"Well," I said, "there we are."

"What's your story, Charlie?"

"I was just running for the fun of it," I said, "and after seven miles or so I got tired. The Vietcong can do forty. It's kind of incredible . . ."

My friend asked his friend what *he* thought. He didn't know. I decided that we would all probably get along better if I established myself as a man of property. "That's my car," I said, pointing.

My friend asked to see my license and registration. He walked to the car.

"I guess that's all right," he said in a moment, "but you're parked illegally."

"I'm not even on the street."

Then the driver backed the police car up to where we were standing.

"Aw, let him go," he said.

"He's parked illegally."

"I'll never do it again," I said.

"Don't let me catch you doing that again," my friend said. "And you'd better not run around at night. There are a lot of suspicious people around."

I didn't know if he meant me or him. I decided to ask him about it some other time.

He climbed back into the car.

"Sorry about the mistake, Charlie," he said. "It's just routine."

"That's *per*fectly all right," I said, "*per*fectly all right."

The next day I ran in Battery Kemble Park again. Except for being chased up a tree by a German shepherd, it was uneventful. The canal towpath is the true center for the social life of the long-distance runner.

Fox Island

I was offered a job as assistant counsel to the House Judiciary Committee, but by then I wanted to write fiction. I moved to Iowa to attend the Iowa Writers' Workshop. Two roommates and I rented a farmhouse eight miles out of town for $75 a month. All three of us played on a club soccer team. I remember the pleasure of heading in a goal on a pass from housemate Bobbie Lehrman to beat Grinnell College, but it was the pastoral side of life that was even more inviting and illuminating.

I love the Iowa landscape. The eastern half of the state is not flat, not if you live in it. There are gentle rises and falls to the land, shadows and brightness in the morning and late afternoon. David Plimpton, my other housemate, had wrestled in college and urged me to join him in a little roadwork— "Just once around the block." Iowa is laid out in sections, each section a square mile bordered by east-west and north-south dirt roads, so "around the block" is four miles. In addition to this, Vance Bourjaily, novelist, World War II vet, and faculty member, took me under his wing to teach me pheasant shooting. I had a Labrador retriever whom I taught out of a manual, twenty minutes a day, until I could send him into a field and move him left or right with hand signals. On his own he would look back every minute or so. He was a brilliant dog. His only fault was that whenever I shot he was certain that there was a bird down, often not the case, and it took a very long time to convince him to give up. Meanwhile, the farmers politely looked away. My dog had a vocabulary of more than fifty words, and he finally learned the phrase "I missed."

Our farmer landlord lived on the far side of the section. He occasionally called up to see if one of us could lend a hand. Farmwork (de-horning steers, castrating shoats, loading and unloading hay bales) is interesting and pleasant exercise if you're called on to do it for only three hours. I liked Barney a lot. He worked at a fast pace and was an excellent and efficient teacher. He liked David and me—he named his two stud boars Dave and John. Bobbie was too busy with his other art, playing the piano, to have time for the farm. I think Barney also stuck up for David and me with the neighboring farmers, who were puzzled and a bit put out to see us jogging around the section. All that energy just going to waste. The neighbors eventually gave us permission to hunt in their fields, giving us an additional eight square miles of hunting pheasant and an occasional covey of quail. Between birds during shooting season, a few fish from the creek, and one large snapping turtle (very chewy), our monthly grocery bill was less than the rent. Our heating bill, however, was huge until we got a couple of potbelly stoves. Barney let us saw down the standing deadwood along the creek. "It'll warm you twice, boys—when you cut it and when you burn it."

There were many things to love about Iowa, but after three years I missed the sea. David Plimpton and I were surprised to learn that we'd both been looking at the undulations of the land and imagining they were ocean swells.

By then I was married, and my wife was expecting a baby.

I'd been neurotically reluctant to send out anything I'd written, but it was time to get over that. An instructorship and part-time work on a Senate campaign weren't enough. Luckily I sold three pieces, two to *The New Yorker* and one to *Sports Illustrated*. Before Maud was born—the best thing in a bountiful year—my father-in-law called to say that there was a very small island for sale in Narragansett Bay. He could see it from his house, a large converted barn. He offered to put up some of the money if I could put up some, the remainder to be mortgaged. I think the price was $52,000.

I was feeling flush, and—watch out for too much good luck—cocky. Cocky about writing and cocky about boats.

I'd spent time in small boats. When I was thirteen I canoed over a fair amount of middle Ontario, which was a wilderness then. I'd rowed in a four-oared shell and in fixed-seat rowboats. I don't know why I thought I knew anything about motorboats. The island came with a beat-up sixteen-foot Boston Whaler and an old outboard motor, and the former owner sold us a twenty-four-foot inboard that looked like a lobster boat with ten feet of the stern cut off.

My wife and I moved the wedding presents we'd stored at her parents' house. It took two trips in the Boston Whaler. The next week my wife and baby Maud stayed onshore at the barn while my job was to get the island shipshape. The first trips in the Boston Whaler didn't go well. The cables from the steering wheel to the outboard were reversed so that to go left you turned the wheel right. That resulted in the near miss of a clump of rocks (actually called "The Clump" on the chart). I hoisted the motor up to avoid bumping it on a submerged rock. When I lowered it I pinched one of the steering cables so that, as I soon found out, the boat turned only left. Fortunately, we hit a wave with enough of a bump to shake open a , panel. Behind it there was a large button. The label had worn off, but it turned out to be the kill switch. While we bobbed around I unpinched the steering cable. The left-right problem now seemed minor, but I decided to buy an old rowboat until I got a bit handier with a motorboat. The rowboat was a beauty, and the boatyard owner, who'd built her, sold her for a song. She was too long to use as a dinghy for a sailboat, and there wasn't much call for a wooden skiff that was too long and slender to take an outboard.

I rowed to the island. When I got to the house, something seemed strange. I couldn't tell what at first. I didn't remember unpacking anything, but there was a small pile of wedding presents, a couple of silver-plated whatnots and a cuckoo clock. In the bedroom the mattress had been turned over and lay crossways. It dawned on me that we'd been robbed. By pros, who could tell silver-plated stuff from sterling and who wouldn't take oddities that could be identified.

I made a sketchy inventory and rowed to Wickford Harbor and walked to the police station. Detective Sergeant O'Dell nodded. "There's been a rash of houses robbed, mostly summer houses on the water. They use a fast boat; I don't have a boat. You're on an island. You want my advice, get a big dog."

"I've got a big dog."

"And get a gun."

"I've got a gun."

"Then do what you need to do. Did it look like they got everything?"

"No. There were some boxes that weren't opened."

"What kind of a gun you got?"

"Double-barreled shotgun."

"Let me know if anything happens."

I rowed out and hid the rowboat behind some bushes. I

spent the night in the attic crawl space. I covered the one small window and read by candlelight, shotgun and Labrador by my side. The second night I considered the shotgun. I'd loaded it with #2 shot, good for geese. Might kill a man at twenty yards. I didn't want to kill anyone. I switched to #4 shot, good for pheasant. After reading another chapter, I thought #4 might kill a man at ten yards. I switched to #8, good for quail.

It was a calm night, the bay still and smooth. I heard a motor. I snuffed the candle and went downstairs to look out a window. A small boat, just visible against the flat, moonlit water. No running lights. Either they were out to poach clams from a restricted area or they were my robbers. I told the dog not to bark. "No barking" was part of his fifty-word vocabulary. I started for the small beach. Went back for the shotgun. I was highly alert but not entirely attentive to detail. I stationed myself among the bushes, a stone's throw from the beach. I heard the scrape of the hull, a grunt as someone tilted the outboard up. The Labrador knew "no barking," but that didn't include "no growling." It was low and rumbling. One of the men shone a flashlight.

I was lit up like a soloist onstage. I raised the shotgun to my shoulder.

There was a lot of clattering. Someone banged something, probably a shin on a gunwale. I couldn't see well after they had shone the light. More clattering, then splashing, the hull scraping. Then another noise. I recognized it because I'd made the same mistake. If you put an outboard motor in reverse without clamping it down, it jumps out of the water and makes a whine like a dentist's drill, a dentist's drill the size of a chain saw.

They got squared away and roared off across the bay.

It turned out they'd been avoiding being caught by listening to the police radio. The police would say, "We see their pickup. We'll wait here till they come back." The robbers, hearing this, would go to their other car on the far side of the bay.

The Wickford harbormaster figured this out. He was technically a law-enforcement officer, but his normal duties were to enforce the no-wake rule inside the harbor. He was made for bigger things. He loaded his lever-action 30.30 and went out at night in his launch. He tucked into a cove. After a while he heard a motor, no running lights. He went after them. Perhaps he used his siren. They didn't stop. When he got abeam of their boat, he fired. I heard it was five rounds, from another source ten rounds. Both accounts said he hit their boat at the waterline. She took on a lot of water. The two men raised their hands.

Their usual MO was to drive their haul to a fence within the hour. This time there was enough loot in their boat to get them sent up.

When I went to see Detective Sergeant O'Dell to report my brief encounter, he grimaced. He said, "Here's what I didn't know last time I talked to you. The harbormaster says they each had a .45 automatic. But what the hell. Sounds like they figured you got the drop on them."

"The dog helped. I've never heard him growl like that."

"Probably picked up on your nerves."

The general wisdom, confirmed by Detective Sergeant O'Dell, was that now that the weather was warming up, the summerhouses would be occupied, there'd be more traffic on the bay, and, of course, the robbers had been caught in a dramatic and widely talked-about way, so that all in all, the citizenry could be confident that piracy had been stamped out on Narragansett Bay.

It turned out the robbery was a windfall. My wife had a list of the wedding presents. Although it was now harder to write thank-you notes with a straight face, the insurance company paid more than we would've got if we'd hocked them.

"Oro mo Bhaidin"

I've loved small boats for as long as I can remember. Canoes first. Then rowboats—not all, not stubby dinghies, not flat-bottomed flat-faced johnboats, but boats that look as though they can move gracefully under oars. I love the flare and curve from bow to waist, the curve and tuck from waist to stern. On calm water I like to hear the rustling of the wake, the sound of the oar blades chinking in. In swells I love the way she lifts and settles, fitting herself to the water.

When I lived on a small island and rowed a flat-iron skiff (prettier than the name), seals would come up to her. They didn't like the sound of motors but were attracted to a musical sound. I'd be rowing along and suddenly see the face of a seal pop up and peer over the transom. Just looking.

I liked being able to do what fishermen in motorboats couldn't do—row through a field of submerged rocks, trolling a spoon for striped bass. I held the rod against the stern thwart with a bare foot, ready to ship the oars and grab the rod if a fish hit the lure.

One night there was a thick fog on the bay. I was woken up by voices on the south side of the island. I pulled on some shorts and went to look. A large motor yacht had bumped into the shore. The man at the wheel was looking around help-lessly. When he saw me he said, "Where the hell am I?"

"Fox Island."

He came out of the wheelhouse and held out a map. It was a road map of southern New England.

I said, "It's a small island, but it shows up on more detailed charts. But look—there's a lot of rocks on this side. Keep her in neutral and I'll push you around to the west side. No rocks."

His wife jumped in, and we pushed and pulled the boat around to just off the bit of sandy beach. I told him the com-pass course to the Wickford breakwater. He looked confused and tired. He said, "I can't see a damn thing in this fog. And the compass keeps doing funny things. Maybe you could come along."

"But how would I get back?" My skiff was pulled up on the beach. I said, "You can follow me."

I propped my flashlight up near the stern and rowed; he and his thirty-five-foot yacht followed the light the two miles and some to Wickford Harbor, his engine going *pocket-a, pocket-a.* I rowed the skiff as fast as I could, close to her top hull speed, a tad over four miles an hour. I figured that if I'd rowed around to my motorboat and got her off the mooring, that whole trip would've been almost as long as it had taken to row. And I wouldn't have been able to hear him if he wanted to say anything. And okay, I was showing off.

When we got to the harbor I did say, "This part of the bay can be confusing."

He said, "Ever think of leaving a light on? So people would know there's an island."

His wife was embarrassed. She said, "Thank you, thank you. You're a regular good old Saint Bernard dog."

He said, "I meant, maybe the government ought to."

I said to her, "I should have tied a flask of brandy around my neck."

"Oh, we don't need any more of *that*."

I didn't want to get in the middle of where this was going. I said to him, "There's the marina. Where the light is. There's a couple of empty slips."

She said to her husband, "You should offer him something."

"No, please don't. I love rowing. Truly." I said it as a hurried politeness, the politeness lost in the hurry.

But halfway back to the island, feeling the skiff glide, watching the bit of line trailing straight off her stern, hearing nothing but her and the oars in the fog silence, I thought there was nowhere I'd rather be, nothing else I'd rather be doing. Truly.

The Watch That Ends the Night
(Outward Bound)

Island living would have been harder had I not met Lenny Chesney. He was on the south side of the island, standing in the water waist-deep, digging up quahogs. I went down to talk with him. He was a sinewy man with white hair tied behind into a short ponytail. He looked like an eighteenth-century American colonial. It turned out we were both talkers, but it also turned out that he was a very good teacher. Over that summer and the next few years he taught me how to dig clams, both long-neck and short-neck; how to catch striped bass, bluefish, flounder, tautog, squeteague; how to bait a lobster pot; how to skin an eel; how to find the island at night in a pea-soup fog. "When you're about to set out, get a compass bearing, check the wind. Set a course for the lee of your island. Let out a line—use about fifteen feet of your white nylon. You'll be rowing, so you can keep an eye on it. If it's straight, you're going straight. You'll feel the wind on your cheek. When you don't, you're in the lee of your island, and you're pretty much there."

When I screwed something up, like forgetting to wire

the eyebolt on the shackle to the mushroom anchor, he'd twist his mouth and say, "Not very salty today, John."

I got a magazine assignment—go take the Outward Bound course at Hurricane Island, Maine. I agreed. My wife and Maud would go to her parents' house; Lenny said he'd keep an eye on the island. I thought twenty-six days in a thirty-foot open boat off the coast of Maine would make me salty. An open boat at sea with ten oarsmen. We'd be Vikings. To get ready I rowed more, swam more, scythed a path around the edge of the island and ran laps.

It turned out to be an experience with more dimensions than saltiness.

PROLOGUE

The first Outward Bound school was established at Aberdovey in Wales in 1941 to help reduce the alarming loss of young British sailors on merchant ships following sinkings by German U-boats. Lawrence Holt, head of the Blue Funnel Line, had noted that while younger and physically better-equipped men succumbed, the older and more experienced officers and petty officers survived. From this he reasoned that success in meeting a severe challenge depends even more on attitude than it does on physical prowess. The educational problem, then, was not so much the recognition of a weakness in the younger men as it was the provision of training situations through which the student could learn to rely on himself to build those qualities of resolution and resilience necessary for survival . . . The Aberdovey Sea School more than fulfilled the hopes of its founders. Graduates of the course held out against adversity at sea, and loss of life diminished . . .

The observable successes of the original programs have led to the extension of Outward Bound into a worldwide twenty-four-school network. Five of these schools are located in the continental United States. Hurricane Island, however, is the only sea school of the five. "We confront ninety-six young men, half of whom are on full scholarship, with the demands of an unfriendly environment."

PETER O. WILLAUER
Director, Hurricane Island Outward Bound School

• ◆ •

FIRST REACTION:
I AM THE VERY MODEL OF
A MODERN MAJOR-GENERAL

There were moments during the Outward Bound course I went through when I was stopped short. Looking back on those moments, I can still feel their keenness. What all those moments had in common—various as they were—was the sense I had of being opened up, of being more alive. I didn't think that that could happen to me in a program whose stated purpose is to give its students that very sense.

In fact, I'd generally found group activities (writers' con-

ferences, Boy Scouts, peace rallies, hootenannies, basic training) to bring out the dullest in everyone. Intelligence lowered
to the lowest common denominator, as in Army basic training. General self-conscious and self-congratulatory babble, as
at fund-raising after-dinner speeches. Cloying sentiments to
which everyone subscribes in bright chirps, or resigned silence.

The first day of Outward Bound was a drag. Rattletrap
buses from Boston to Rockland, Maine. My bus seemed to
have a fair number of college jocks. Track, soccer, swimming.
There was a lot of comparing notes on good workouts with
weights. *Fine,* I thought. *That's what I'm here for. Some high-class
competition to pull me out of the slough of young middle age.* There
was also some nervous chatter about what was in store for us.

"Jeez—fifty yards underwater. I don't know if I can make
that." Speaker flexing abnormally developed pecs. Obvious
mock modesty.

"Fifty yards? That's just two lengths of a pool. It's a question
of hyperventilation." Second speaker meeting mock-modesty
ploy with breezy confidence gambit.

Further discussion of sailing, rowing, rock climbing, six-
mile run.

"How fast do they make you run?" Note use of impersonal
they.

Breezy confidence speaker: "The six miles? It's a *race,* isn't it?"

"No. I mean, every morning before breakfast. They couldn't
just wear you right out in the morning, could they?" *They.*

All that bus-ride talk seems distant and irrelevant now. As
does the ex-marine who met us on the pier in Rockland—
complete with surplus campaign hat, surplus fatigues, surplus
command voice, and surplus hard stare at raw recruits. (In all
fairness, he was atypical, and that was his worst moment.)

We were divided up into watches (crews of twelve) and

boarded the ferry, which made its way off into a cold fog. *Pea soup* not the word. *Cod-liver-oil aspic.* Our watch a "senior" watch. Average age twenty-eight. By far the most sedate. Official name of our watch Slocum (after Joshua), but we were soon called the Geritol watch. Other watches more colorful. Several boys with shoulder-length ringlets. One gold earring. Several shaved heads. A lot of institutional sweatshirts of colleges, schools, and athletic clubs. One cowboy outfit. Our only bit of dash was Johnny Cora, a black Puerto Rican who looked as though he'd just stepped out of Sunny's Gym to do his roadwork. He was in fact an ex-boxer, now a social worker. The rest of our watch looked like a weekend in the backyard. A couple of teachers, a psychologist, another social worker, four college seniors, one ex–Peace Corpsman, one seminarian about to become a priest, and me.

First surprise on Hurricane Island: our watch officer, Jed Williamson, introduced us to our assistant watch officer. It was his wife, Perry. We dumped our gear in two six-man platform tents and set off on a tour of the island. At a trot. Up and down rocky trails, through lush spruce woods. Several of our watch winded. Gentlemanly impulse to help Perry (who is quite elegantly pretty) over the rocks checked. She wasn't breathing hard.

Group discussion on rock by sea. A few words on why we thought we were there. We each introduced someone else to the group. Reminiscent of the first day of a freshman English course at a midwestern university. A few embarrassing effusions—"I think Mike sounds like a really interesting member of the group"—but, naturally enough, most people playing cards close to their chests.

More jogging. Then first "initiative test." Problem: move entire group from one large tree to another large tree—fifteen or twenty yards—without touching the ground in between. Hanging from a rope stretched between the trees were—in order—a rope, three tires, and another rope. All of them were just far enough apart so that an average person couldn't quite reach the next tire or rope without either getting a push from behind or having the tire or rope in front swung back toward him. The first rope was too far from the starting line to leap at, but there was a two-by-four provided to use in any way we wanted. We used it to snag the first rope. If it or anyone touched the ground, it or he was "out," no longer available for use, "reduced to ashes by chemically treated pine needles between the trees." Ho, ho, ho. Jed pulled out his pocket watch and said it should take ten minutes.

Without much talk we launched ourselves. The first guy pulled the rope back with the two-by-four and swung to tire one. The second guy bumped him from tire one to tire two. But soon we somehow had people stranded on all three tires. They were more unstable than they looked. The problem was that the tires kept spinning, so that if you tried to pump yourself, as on a swing, there was no way of knowing which way your thrust would take you. Actually, that was only the technical problem. The *problem* was chaos. I thought at the time that a contributing cause of the chaos was that no one wanted to point out to someone who was being inept that he was inept, and in what way he was inept. A not-altogether-sound conclusion.

Jed commented that for all the assembled brawn and brains it was an amazingly bad performance. Some people felt cast down by that. I didn't feel very hangdog; we'd had a good time. We jogged off to pick up equipment—seaboots, foul-weather gear, hooded sweatshirt and sweatpants, sleeping bag, plastic tarp, mess kit, rigging knife, life jacket, and whistle.

Later in the course there were some mumblings about the gear. The sleeping bags were not quilted goose down. Some of the seaboots leaked. The foul-weather gear and life jackets were superb, however. All in all, I think it a wise decision to provide the equipment there. Otherwise there would be some people showing up in hundred-dollar seagoing outfits and others showing up with see-through plastic galoshes that would dissolve the first time they touched a barnacle-covered rock. It's already enough that rich kids usually have sailed before and that poor kids usually haven't. That can be overcome. By the end of some of the four- and five-day expeditions it does happen that a guy who hasn't seen water bigger than a bathtub is at the helm, holding a compass course on a foggy heaving sea while the members of the Suburbia Yacht Club are bringing up breakfast over the lee rail. But basic equipment isn't a matter of will or learning, so the school lays it on.

That evening we all signed a "pledge" in a rather somber ceremony in the mess hall. For the duration of the twenty-six days we were not to smoke (anything) and not to drink alcohol, and we undertook to "live in good fellowship." That sounds rather Boy Scoutish, but it was unpretentious, actually, and turned out to have interesting consequences.

We retired to our tents through the fog. That is, most of us retired to our tents. There were at least a dozen lost sheep in the darkness who wandered forlornly up rocks, through woods, into puddles. Occasionally one would find our tent, poke his head through the flaps, and say, "Hey—you in my watch?"

"What watch are you in?"

"Nansen."

"Oh. You're on top of that hill, I think; just jog up the hill." But he'd be back. As the night wore on, the conversations with the intruding heads grew less helpful. The lost sheep seemed more like stray dogs.

"Hey. Anyone here from Nansen?" No answer from the night.

"Hey. Naaan-seeeennnn!" No answer. Foghorn on Heron Neck moaned. Sound of trampling through bushes. Muffled voice: "Sheee-it."

I suppose for a lot of guys it was the first time without lights since the New York blackout.

After perhaps an hour there were no more stragglers. However, there was the sound of a voice we were to come to know well. Probably the youngest boy of the whole group was in the tent across the trail from us. At one a.m. he was still yakking nervously. His voice had the same fog-penetrating quality as the Heron Neck horn.

"Hey . . . Hey. You asleep? Like hell you were. Hey. What kind of cigarettes you giving up? Jeez, what I'd give for a smoke." Et cetera, et cetera. Irritating but poignant. He didn't want to be alone.

By two-thirty the only sound was the Heron Neck horn. I walked down to the latrine and back. I was half amazed (what insanity had brought me here?), half lulled by the surrounding spruce and fog.

Up at five-thirty. By five-thirty-five most of us running in place to keep warm while we waited for late risers. Off for our run by five-thirty-eight. Easy pace, for which I was grateful. I'd done something painful to a rib cartilage two weeks before and hadn't done any exercise since then. It had hurt to breathe at all for a week, and still hurt to breathe deeply. We worked up a lather and then jumped into the quarry pool. That was a first-day luxury. After that we jumped into the sea. Much colder. But the first day was cozy—the fog hid the cliff that rose on one side of the pool. It also hid the fact that there were about a hundred of us running in groups of twelve. We ran and swam in a fifty-foot circle of visibility.

It was the second day when we had our first class in seamanship and navigation. I say "class" guardedly. Perhaps I should say "lesson." We were taken down to a whaleboat. The basic classroom of the school. Thirty feet long. Seven feet wide in the very middle. Pointed at both ends. A big lifeboat, really. We got in. Five rowing benches to seat ten rowers. Another man at the helm and one on bow watch. One of the school's lobster boats took us in tow. No fog. Bright, pure weather with a fresh breeze. We sat back and watched the water froth past. Gulls and cormorants. Attractive rocky islands. We skipped between islands, around islands, past islands. We were settling into promenade-deck lounge-chair amiability when we stopped. As the lobster boat surged off in an irritating display of power a voice called back, "Lunch is at twelve-thirty."

First lesson in seamanship and navigation. We broke out the oars and the rudder. So far, so good. Some people have tried rowing ten oars without a rudder. I don't think they've got back in time for lunch. We'd also kept track of the zigs and zags, so all we had to do was row. We rowed. It was awful.

I like rowing. One of my hopes for the program had been to set out with a band of stalwart Vikings manning the sweeps. It hadn't occurred to me till then that someone wouldn't know how to row. It seemed to me more basic and easier than riding a bicycle. Yet half of our crew couldn't handle an oar. Some dipped the blades in three feet deep. A few missed the water altogether. For ten minutes we floundered, the blades cracking against one another or slicing deep into the water, surfacing unexpectedly to tangle with the oar in front. I felt a deep aesthetic wound.

There were a few mild murmurings.

"Do you think you could avoid hitting me in the back?"

"Shouldn't we keep together?"

My wounded sensibility cried out "Yes," and I became, I cringe to admit it, a "take-charge guy." My speech was not a frenzy of perfection. I didn't suggest feathering, for example. I mentioned using more muscle than just the arms, how deep the blade should go in the water, and the importance of rhythm.

We set off again. A moment of improvement and then exasperation. All but one or two were doing passably, and so it seemed to me that those persisting in error must not be trying. It also seemed to me that I scarcely said more than to occasionally croak a cadence. "Stroke—and forward together—stroke—recover together and—stroke . . ."

We got back to the island by the end of the morning. Twelve-twenty, to be exact. But mooring the boat and running to the dining hall took fifteen minutes, and we found ourselves locked out from lunch. That was a minor irritation compared to the shattering of my dream voyage in which "the shining oars smote the wine-dark sea."

We scattered along the shore to eat raspberries. When we met back at the tents I was still in a rage of disappointment and frustration. I'd been ready to be asked to dare sturdy feats of rowing. To set out across the Gulf of Maine. "It may be we shall touch the Happy Isles." And we couldn't even get back for lunch.

During the ensuing group discussion I held my tongue. Question on the floor was: Why had we moved so slowly?

Answers: Too much time spent explaining. (*Ha!* I thought, *Too much time dragging your oar under the boat.*) Maybe there was too much insistence on perfection right away. (*Ha! You spent half the time hitting people in the back and the other half looking for your gloves because you had a tiny blister.*)

After these opinions had been ventured, by the most bungling rower, naturally, there was a strained silence. I ventured what I thought was a restrained version of my feelings, cloaked in quasi-apology: "I'm sorry if I may have seemed—uh—overbearing. However, I think it should be clear that if you want your oar to go into the water in rhythm, it must *leave* the water in rhythm, and recover in rhythm. Of course," I went on resignedly, "it may just take time until everyone gets it down."

Bungling rower: "You don't have to do all that to row. There aren't any bad rowers here."

I am surprised I could have been taking this all so seriously. Especially since I couldn't have been more loose about the initiative tests. I am also surprised at the isolation that irritation can bring. During the row back (I was rowing stroke), I was aware of every oar that entered the water late or early. That was all that was on my mind about every person in the boat.

From Loong-Ho Tan, our Chinese Malay exchange student from Brandeis: "If it is necessary—to accomplish a task—to follow an overbearing one, I for one will gladly swallow my pride and follow if it be necessary to the task."

My thoughts of the moment, if not exactly. I noticed that he referred to an "overbearing one." I had used the word in apologetic self-deprecation, in polite exaggeration of a fault in myself that I described to myself as "slight impatience."

We went off for another try at the swinging-tire initiative test. We figured it out. And so off to the wall and the beam. The next several days were pleasantly rigorous. Morning run for two and a half miles. Jump into sea. Rowing peapods. Sailing the whaleboat rigged with spritsails. We also rowed it. There was the ropes course (walking across a log suspended by ropes, stepping to another log suspended by ropes three feet below, up a rope ladder, across a beam to a Burma bridge, around a treetop to another single-strand bridge with only one other rope hand high to steady with, down a rope to a tippy steel hammock strung between trees, up a tree to a swinging rope, swing across to a cargo net, et cetera). We learned "drownproofing," which is a way of floating like a jellyfish to conserve energy. You breathe only every thirty or forty-five seconds. Once you get into the rhythm it tends to relax you so much that you feel as if you're dissolving in the water. You can actually float and even propel yourself around with your feet and hands tied.

We had a preliminary lesson in rock climbing—knots and belaying procedures. Also navigation. And at the end of the day we would sometimes do circuit training, a variety of timed exercises, usually a dozen exercises for two minutes each. Jed had a quasi-medical interest in testing normal pulse rates, exertion pulse rates, and five-minute recovery rates. By the end of the course my normal pulse rate dropped, my exertion rate stayed the same (although I was exerting more), and my recovery rate was almost back to normal. I would guess that Jed's interest in pulse rates dates from the time he spent on the U.S. biathlon team. I imagine that the target-shooting parts would be quite difficult if your pulse was throbbing away at 160 or so.

We also had a session of ecology in preparation for being marooned on a bare island. The word *ecology,* like the phrase *seamanship and navigation,* is used in its most practical sense. What you can eat. Armed with our Euell Gibbons pamphlets on "eating wild," we roamed the shore tasting orache, sow thistle, rose hips, and sheep sorrel. Our instructor in ecology was a very demure British guy from Australia. When they're British down there, they're more British than the British. As we wandered along I heard him say, "Oh, I shouldn't eat any more of those if I were you. One or two won't do any harm, but you'll feel quite awful if you persist."

"What are they?"

"Deadly nightshade."

This week of training may sound as though it's totally related to the physical. And it's true that getting up at five-thirty in the morning and being more or less violently active until sunset meant that shortly after dark nearly everyone had collapsed in his bunk. I had no problem with insomnia. But there was a less obvious side effect—a mute cohesion of the group. We politely vied with one another for the less pleasant cleaning details ("I'll wash out the urinals"—"No, let me do it, you did it last time"). There was a lull in whatever strains there had been. There was also a blunting of curiosity about where people came from, and what they did. As I recall, there was even a change in the faces—a relaxation of mannerisms and tics. The people in our watch all seemed to have slightly dreamy, earnest expressions. Not forced; in fact, unconscious. José—coincidentally, another black Puerto Rican who'd done some boxing—was probably the most restless, but that was intermittent.

One evening at supper we asked if we could just walk around the island. We'd been completely around it only while running, and we hadn't really looked at more than roots, puddles, and footholds in the rocks. We all walked up to a headland on the west side. We all sat down. A hundred feet below, swells were squeezing into the sound between Hurricane Island and

Little Hurricane. The swells were tripped up by a ledge and combed over the rocks in mid-channel. The sun turned red behind a strip of clouds. I'd been a little wary of a group setting out to Be Still Together, but I felt an undeniable easing of the spluttering and crackling silence that goes on between people who happen not to be talking. It's usually like static on an open line, but we'd not only stopped transmitting—we'd turned off the whole phone system. It was very comfortable.

A herring gull started to patrol the water, a hundred feet above the sea, eye level with us. He went a hundred yards into the wind without moving a feather, then wheeled and floated downwind. After a hundred yards he came about neatly and soared upwind, still not moving his wings but not losing a foot of altitude, intent on the surge of water below us. He glided back and forth for fifteen minutes or so—I have no idea of the time, really, except that the sun had set when he flew off, and when we climbed down the hillside and walked home along the shore.

From that time on I felt an affection for the island and its waters and life that none of the things that happened later diminished.

•◆•

THE WATCH THAT ENDS THE NIGHT

We set off on our first expedition on a gray day with a stiff breeze. Perry didn't come along, much to everyone's disappointment. Instead, we took along a severe Australian salt. As he was coming down with a mysterious summer flu, his Captain Bligh moods outstripped mine by several lengths. I had been elected captain, but whatever mild command I gave was usually overwhelmed by raucous Aussie cries.

"Harden in on those sails! Are you listening? Are you awake? Wakey, wakey, wakey! You're not *sailing,* you 'orrible men."

But it was good sailing. The boat moved surprisingly easily through the chop. The more it blew, the more graceful she became. It was nice to think of her being transformed by the wind from the slow barge we'd rowed back late for lunch into this white-winged bird.

That night we camped out on an island near the north end of North Haven. Johnny Cora and I spent the night on board as anchor watch. The next day the wind died at noon (usually when it came up). We rowed. The sea like glass. Much improved rowing. Just beyond our blades a porpoise rolled its back. I'd seen porpoises from ships and in aquariums—this was much more exciting. No distance, no captivity. Being at sea like this was what I'd dreamed of. Glistening porpoises, and later on a seal. The islands were barren but inviting.

Unfortunately, we had some disagreement about where we'd stop for supper. The staff was for pushing on and the crew was for picking an easy mark. Our whole trip was nothing much but an extended circumnavigation of Vinalhaven and North Haven, and the farther north we went, the farther we'd have to go to get home. Our Australian instructor's virus settled into his intestine, and that settled the discussion, too. We pulled for the evening rendezvous with the other whaleboats. When we finally anchored for supper we were all a bit dingo from the sun. Couldn't get sense out of anyone. We lay about in this state until the other boats showed up. After supper we learned that we weren't spending the night there. We were to get some practice traveling at night.

At about ten we were simultaneously beset by swarms of mosquitoes and a chilling wind. The mosquitoes were extremely hardy. I thought it abnormal and unfair that we had cold and bugs together.

As soon as we pushed off in convoy, however, the wind died to a whisper. We rowed with our sails up, keeping in touch with the other boats by flashing a light on our mainsail from time to time. Our running lights were kerosene lanterns that wouldn't stay lit.

The wind picked up to a murmur, and we pulled the oars in. As soon as they were boated, the rowers collapsed in place into huddled sleep. I'd been off the helm all day so that everyone would get a chance. I scuttled back to relieve the helmsman, who promptly curled up like a spider beside the first rower. Jed and I passed a few words about the night (moonless), the course (187), and insomnia. The word jerked me awake. "I don't have insomnia," Jed said. "I just don't sleep much." But he pulled himself into a tight *N* in the stern sheets and dozed off.

The next hour was deeply, deeply satisfying. I was the only one awake, the boat a communal cradle gliding placidly toward a star, conveniently on course. Not a sound but the sighs of twelve sleepers and the water bubbling slowly past our stern.

We landed on Saddle Island at four in the morning, left an anchor watch, and crashed up a hill into the underbrush. Everyone was spent. Some of us lay down without sleeping bags. José, with whom I'd packed my gear, pulled me and our duffel and his friend Johnny up the hill into a mossy spot between two shelves of granite. Just as we got our sleeping bags unrolled, another boat from the convoy arrived. They shoehorned their boat in beside ours, filling the cove with curses that echoed up the hillside. A tiny auxiliary cruising sloop that was anchored nearby hoisted her anchor and putt-putted away. Our hillside was very small, mostly rocks and bushes, but the invaders came on, holding their duffels in front of their faces to keep from being lashed by branches, and still swearing away, as though they were trying to find their way by sonar. Their watch officer, a rather nice prep-school English teacher, found his way into our nook. From there he lectured his crew on what a crummy thing they'd done in driving the sloop away. Since the crew avoided him, this had the beneficial by-product of saving us from being trampled. I was lulled to sleep by his voice.

The next sound I heard was the hum of mosquitoes at dawn. But oddly enough, we all felt fresh after less than two hours' sleep. I discussed this with several of our watch who were as amazed as I was.

We rowed and sailed all morning until by lunch we were almost back at Hurricane Island. We didn't go there, however. The convoy split up after lunch, each boat dumping its crew on a small island. Jed explained that this was "group solo." He gave me some matches, two plastic sheets, and two #10 cans. We were left without any other gear. So that the twelve of us wouldn't strip the island of everything edible, we'd been left a side of mutton.

This exercise was irritating in that we were almost "home"— to wit, tents, bunks, showers, hot coffee, and our usual gorge of food. From the cliffs at one end of our "group solo" island we could actually see Hurricane Island—in fact, the very spot where we'd sat to watch the herring gull patrol his waters. But we'd been told it was just for another twenty-four hours, and everyone was cheerful, as the sun was shining.

I was still "captain," but there was very little to direct that

I could see. I was wrong again, as it turned out. We were, as always, allowed to build our fire only in a #10 can, which meant that cooking had to be done in small portions in the other can. We had the services of a good trail cook from Alaska—Rod, our senior colleague (he never did tell his real age, but it was certainly forty). He worried the meat into gobbets, and the rest of us gathered twigs for the fire and edible greens for the stew. We had mussels for a starter.

I gave one plastic sheet to Rod and the other to Loong-Ho on the theory that they had the least body fat. I went off and built a lean-to and nest of branches, leaves, and brown spruce boughs.

Almost everyone froze that night. Rod gave his plastic sheet to Dave, who rolled up in it beside the fire, which Rod fed twigs every twenty minutes. In spite of the cold, the mosquitoes were out in force.

What I should have done, I learned much later, was to get everyone together under both plastic sheets to keep warm in a sort of body pod. Instead of Rod staying up to keep the fire smoldering for only a few people, we could have set up shifts to keep it glowing with dry sticks for warmth and smoking with green twigs as a smudge pot. In addition, the person on fire watch could have waved a spruce bough as a fly-and-mosquito whisk over all our heaped bodies. Mistake number four was that we kept our foul-weather gear on, and the moisture that had been steaming around all day without a chance of escaping wet our clothes through and conducted away our body heat until we felt like wet lettuce at the bottom of the icebox. A miserable night for all, for which I felt I was to blame. My impulse had been to burrow in my own hole far away.

Still, the island was an extremely attractive one when the sun came up again. Massive granite cliffs on the side open to the sea. A high crown of spruce and hardwood, with oddly tidy clearings of bright emerald grass. We collected a couple of rock crabs, some mussels, and a potful of greens for breakfast and then wandered off for naps in the clearings or on the rocks.

I had my first long conversation in two weeks that day. With Pat—one of the several remarkable people in our watch. Earnest—zealous—but reasonable about a number of things, including politics and law. Swimmer, skier, runner. His sister had been through the Minnesota Outward Bound school; his brother was currently at the Colorado Outward Bound school. "We're a family of fanatics," he said pleasantly. He very quickly picked up rowing and sailing and climbing, none of which he'd done before, but his eye was quite rightly on something beyond. It was not just that he had a refined experimental approach to his own experiences, but he was also very alert to the positions that people found themselves in in the watch and *their* view of the situation. He himself had a much more deliberate and functional view of the other people than I had—I tended to clutter up my ideas with hypotheses beyond the plain facts.

It was comforting to know that the whole boat and crew were sensed and appreciated—in short, *existed* in someone else's brain in clearly observed form.

Back to Hurricane Island that evening. Hot shower. Looked in steamy mirror over washbasin. Expected to find outward and visible signs of inward and spiritual grace of past two weeks. Same old mug. Only a remarkable mound of mosquito bites on forehead—felt like a pile of dried peas.

We went on duty watch the next day. Duties—monitoring the radios (the school sends out rescue parties if called), checking the generator and the water pumps, and helping in the kitchen. I happened to see an outward and visible sign then.

The watch we relieved had just got back from ten days in their whaleboat (they had a slightly different program from ours) and were about to go home. They had, as a group, a most extraordinary presence. It was partly that they were brimming with farm-boy-on-Saturday-night energy—stored raw sun and an urge to *do* something. But it was also the way they treated one another. They were being very breezy all around, as though they'd been going out in their whaleboat for years and years, and liking it and one another more and more. I realized that in our group, all our docility and care with one another meant that we were still very wary and able to be offended, and I couldn't imagine that another two weeks would make much difference. But it was still a pleasure to see this crew lolling about happily in their seaboots, laughing about this or that that had happened to them at sea. The light leaking out of the rescue tent caught the glossy patches of their oilskins and the white of their teeth and eyes. Like Rembrandt's painting of the night watch, I knew I was off on a romantic tangent, but why not?

•◆•

AND CAST ADOWN THE PROUD

The next couple of days we spent mostly climbing the cliff rising out of the quarry. For some insane reason I thought I wanted to get right into it. I volunteered to go first on climb number three. Careless exuberance? Ambition to be top dog?

From the first move I realized this was going to be paralyzing. It wasn't like anything I'd ever done. I'd caught a whiff of fear on the ropes course, and I'd seen one of us struck immobile with fear. I had felt pity, not sympathy.

I suppose what we were doing would be called technical rock climbing. It required not just a certain strength or just balance. It required both, plus calm foresight and cunning. I leaked out all my calm foresight and cunning after three or four moves up and one look down. One problem was that I couldn't get used to not resting. Once you were on the cliff there was no point in stopping, because you were always tiring out something just holding on—hands, ankles, knees, back. Second, I tended to forget about the belay. It was erased from my deep thoughts. If someone had asked me what would happen if I fell I could have answered after some reflection, "Oh— I'm on a belaying rope. I won't go all the way down." But I derived no comfort from this information. It was nothing for my fears (vivid pictures of my body splattering on a rock, being impaled on a dead tree limb) to latch onto.

A third difficulty was that it was impossible to move with a burst of nerve and energy to the next spot, because the next spot would be, for example, a narrow ledge on which you balanced more than stood. You couldn't arrive in a rush.

The last difficulty I'll mention—the list is actually quite long—was that I couldn't calm down. My breathing was so shallow it barely got past my back molars.

By the time I got two-thirds of the way up the cliff I was really weak in the knees. I'd heard nothing since I began from the climbing instructor who was belaying me—a jovial and muscular Englishman named Bill Aughten. I couldn't see him on account of an overhang. I called up in a weak voice to ask if he was still there and knew my life was still in his hands.

"*My* hands, is it?" he said. "I'd hate to think that."

"I mean, you've got me belayed?"

"Belayed? Well, I've got a bit of rope around a bit of a twig, and I *assume* it goes on down to you. In fact, I'm *almost* sure of it. Just come along, then . . ."

Oddly enough, this vaudeville encounter was just right. It gave me a burst of energy that arose out of slight irritation, a desire to impress and even one-up Aughten with a nonchalance of my own, and a certain reassurance—I mean, he wouldn't *dare* kid around if things weren't going okay.

There was one artificial device on this climb. I was just beneath a short rope that hung over the overhang. I got a hand on it and then, abandoning my one toehold, got another hand on it. I moved my feet up, soles flat against the wall. The trick now was to run to the left and then back to the right as fast as one could and then swing like a pendulum. At the end of the arc to the right there was a ledge. One was expected to let go of mother rope (so solid, so graspable) and get the palms of one's hands onto the ledge and then hoist one's torso up (called *mantling*) until it was possible to get a foot up and stand. The ledge was the size of the arm of an armchair.

I made all three moves in a haze of faith, imitating by dim memory what Aughten had done when he'd gone up. I had the dim memory only because it was a pretty flashy maneuver. It wasn't as hard as it looked (unlike almost every other move on the face). I got to the ledge and mantled up. A few more moves and I was on top. I crawled away from the edge of the cliff on all fours. I was sure I'd be drawn over the edge by some mysterious force. I undid the double figure-eight knot tied in the belaying rope from the carabiner in my waistband and moved away from the edge another five feet. Aughten said in a kindly way, "It's a good thing you didn't scratch around too badly. It always unnerves the others when the first student makes a hash of it."

But no triumph. No comfort. I saw no joy in rock climbing. I was shaken. By the time I got to my feet, another guy appeared. He was jubilant. He'd loved it. He'd been challenged, terrified, and relieved to get to the top, but he felt as though he'd won a game. I didn't. I felt as though an evil spirit had sucked three pints of my blood.

We all tried some more climbs. I scratched and heaved up one that by all accounts was easier than the one I'd started with. We tapered off the day by fooling around with walking up a steep rock slope and trying to jump up and catch a ledge with one hand and then grab a higher ledge with the other hand. No sense of danger in these. Just hard exercise.

Everyone else got better, though, and I got worse. It was partly a question of exuberance. Theirs grew; mine shrank. I dreaded the next day of rock climbing.

•◆•

Early in the morning. Overcast. We watched Paul Ross, the other climbing instructor, make the climb. It was impressive. He looked great. Apparently, he's quite famous in climbing circles. Even I could tell he was stylish. No artificial help over the overhang on his climb. As soon as he'd done it I forgot what he'd done. I didn't volunteer to go first. I wanted to, but by the time a noise came out of my mouth a half-dozen others had volunteered.

At last I started to climb. I moved more and more slowly, to just under the overhang. I'd felt more and more muddled with each move. A great weight on my limbs and mind. Even before I fell I was humiliated. An accumulation of frustration and defeated resignation was all I had in my head when I tried to move up the overhang. I couldn't hear anything, although apparently Bill Aughten was giving me advice. I got a hand on the top of the overhang. I somehow got my head up above it, too. I could see Bill Aughten's lips moving. I moved my other hand up. There was no place to hold. Only smooth rock, too steep to mantle on. My toes were slipping against the face underneath the overhang. I knew it was all wrong, but I couldn't think. I felt a wedge of air slide between my chest and the overhang. Very slowly. It didn't occur to me to grab the belaying rope. As it turned out, it was so slack I would have spilled off anyway. I knew it was bad form to clutch the rope (which is supposed to be a safety device of last resort). I had forgotten about it. The wedge of air squeezing me off the cliff swelled. My fingers slid across the top of the overhang, filing my nails short. My feet, receiving my weight for an instant, held firm. Then my weight vanished altogether. I looked deep into the receding gray sky. Until I was caught by the rope on my waistband.

Nylon rope will stretch half its length under strain. With that bit of elastic bounce I may have fallen fifteen feet. I dangled like a spider on its thread for a bit and then was lowered all the way to the ground. I'd been almost at the top.

"Are you going to try again?" Perry asked.

"Yes," I said, but automatically.

It occurred to me that even before I began my last effort I had given up. I had allowed myself so much panicky muddle that I had thrashed around like a horse who's frightened blind by a spill. I had foreseen the spill and been frightened into it. I tried to work backward through my feelings, trying to leave fright and humiliation for useful rage. I overshot it and ended up in numbness again.

"I'll go up again if nobody minds," I said to Perry experimentally.

"Sure," she said. "No one minds, except maybe Bill Aughten. It can give you a terrific rope burn to catch someone falling like *that*."

That perked me up. I couldn't tell out of what feeling that remark emerged. It may have been a pedagogical goad. It may have been that my stiffened face didn't show enough concern.

Paul Ross called me over to an easy climb at the end of the cliff. I said I was going up the hard one again. He insisted I get the easy part of the program out of the way. In my state it wasn't easy. Paul talked me up—do this, do that—which was not the standard method. They liked to just let you work it out yourself.

I got to the top and sat around near the third exercise, which was to rappel down the blankest part of the cliff face. It looked fairly easy, from what I'd seen from the bottom. But I didn't get into line. There was a stream of our people coming up the easy route and a few coming up the hard way still. Maybe it would soon be time for us all to quit, I hoped. George, our psychologist, sat down with me for a while. We passed a few remarks about my psychic state. I was clutching my knees, rocking my body, and staring vacantly out to sea. I hadn't done that since the first time I'd been knocked around in a high-school football game. Combination of being bruised, out of breath, and bewildered. George went through his theory that I was reestablishing the rhythm of the womb. He recommended rappelling down as even better therapy than rocking. He was right about that, at least. Rappelling down was great fun. It was like walking backward on the moon.

Started up the hard way again. By the time I got to the overhang I was working hard, but I wasn't in a muddle. I was concentrating. I thought awhile, just calculation, not spasms. I finally thought I knew what to do. Without going into details, I can say: (a) that it is amazing how little grip it takes to keep from falling—I'd been grabbing so hard I was almost pushing myself off; (b) it is equally amazing how much weight the simple friction of your flat soles will bear against the cliff face, even without an actual foothold. All you have to do (all!) is keep your weight pressing down from directly above. A straight line through your center, your feet, and the earth's center.

I was happy to get to the top. I'd learned something concrete. It worked. Bill Aughten, once again forsaking his usual ironic mode, said, "That's quite good—climbing up after falling off in that—ah—thorough way."

Corny jubilation. Fortunately, I didn't say anything. However, I looked over the cliff, and Perry waved up. I blew her a kiss. I rushed off to try a twenty-foot layback—climbing up a four-inch crack in the face by sticking your fingers and toes into it, all close together. José and Loong-Ho made it the first time. Everyone but me made it the second time. Very good for the group. I was again in as much of a muddle as I was when trying to flail over the overhang and slipping off. No third try. I didn't get how to do it. Lump it.

·◆·

SOLO: SONG WITHOUT WORDS

From what I've heard from pilgrims to other Outward Bound schools, Hurricane Island has the most bountiful solo. It has the sea. It does entail being marooned on a small island for four days to fend for yourself. There is a "solo kit": eleven matches, a jug of water, a sleeping bag, a plastic sheet, a tin can to build fires in (actually, a limitation of the fire hazard rather than a help to the survivor), and the clothes one normally wears on the whaleboat.

"What did you eat?" is what people ask. But the primary point of the exercise wasn't finding food. It was an interesting incidental point, but it became less of a point each day. Visions and daydreams were more interesting.

The Plains Indians used to send out their young men to be alone, to fast, and to have dreams—to dream of their totem, the spirit of an animal or plant or some aspect of nature that would then guide them or inspire them and whose reappearance in various guises would be a portent throughout their lives. Needless to say, the Outward Bound solo is not so explicitly spiritual. But there still is supposed to be—explicitly— more to it than learning to fill your belly with roots, leaves, and animal life. In the language of modern counseling the point of the exercise is "to live with yourself," "to face the challenge of an unfamiliar environment."

Of course I'm not sure I can do much better. I have only a little to say about the experiences of the other watch members. When we all got back together, some of the guys said they'd been "going through some heavy changes," but to quiz them about it would have been like hanging around a confessional in a Catholic church, running up to an emerging penitent and saying, "You're in a state of grace, huh? Got all those mortals and venials off your chest? Any juicy ones?"

Much later I learned that one of our watch decided to get married while on solo. It would be a good time to think about getting married. Contrary to what you might think, you're not in a goatlike state of deprivation. In fact, it is a momentary hiatus of strong appetites—sex, food, muscular exertion. I think most people finally just feel clear.

I'd planned to think about a novel I'd written that was somehow askew. I couldn't. Instead, I was very happy to browse on glasswort, sea blite, and goosetongue, and to look at the tide erasing a bright sandbar with an advance that was a model of the earth's monthly shadowing of the moon. The water dwindled the thick strand into a graceful scimitar, then into a thinner and thinner crescent, until it was all awash.

All in all the experience is more Proustian than Joycean. An arrangement of stones under the water, or the smell of the earth, or the feel of your own skin, can embark your senses inward and backward among specimens of surprisingly preserved (but usually inaccessible) times in your memory. I say "rather than Joycean" because it is your senses and then your memory-senses that are stirred directly; the very last thing to come into your head is a word. With Joyce the word often precedes sensing. On the island I often saw—sensed—a swirl of plovers rising from the strand, and what the sight touched off in me was other sights, shorn of names or a place in time.

Of course there is still time left over even after being in Proustian states, thinking of totems, or keeping a Thoreau-like journal. In fact, the truth is that my first day was urgently practical: Looks like rain. Shelter. Where? Scurry around island. Ah. Under large spruce. Windbreak. Which side? Where is prevailing wind? Southwest? Northeast? Where are they? No sun. Guess. Haul driftwood to make windbreak. Rig plastic sheet overhead. Store kindling. Four days! Remember mosquitoes and cold. Four days. Damn. When is low tide? Now? Gather mussels, whelks. Not low enough to reach sea urchins. Gather handful of rose hips for breakfast. Sprinkling of rain. Dig ditch around shelter. Smugness at that shrewd move. Make nest of leaves and grass. Takes forever. Tempted to cut spruce boughs. Resist temptation. More leaves and grass. Tide almost in. Not much time before dark. Boil whelks and mussels. Mussels so-so. Whelks awful. Thank God it's dark so I can't see them. Just pop the whelk in. I'm sure it's writhing around in my mouth. Could it still be alive? Do they resist boiling? It's fighting back at being chewed, lashing its white wormy coils. I chew it in a rage. Die, repulsive whelk! Eat rose hips to get whelk memory out of my mouth. Can't stop with one. Orgy of rose hips. Don my hooded sweatshirt and pull strings so that only my nose is available to mosquitoes. Drowse. Wake in darkness to sound of a rain squall moving across water toward the island. Louder and louder. It passes through spruce. I'm dry. I like the sound.

The rest of solo was timeless. Usually the nature of time is social. Measured by obligations to other people. Work. Lunch. Dinner. Who, when. Here the only events are sunrise, sunset, high tide, low tide.

My best meal was of eight elvers (baby eels) and a tiny green crab. Scooped them up like a bear catching salmon. Also dandelion roots—like small parsnips. The island was stripped of blueberries and raspberries by vacationing cruisers earlier. I was soon tired of greens and mussels. Sea-urchin roe superb, however.

On the last day I met a family from a cruising sloop. My voice sounded funny. Also I was very modest—checked several times to make sure everything was buttoned up before emerging from the bushes onto the beach. Attractive family—all of them. Children helped me shell strand-wheat grains. I felt like a half-tame mangy bear. When they left I was relieved to be alone, not because I didn't relish their company but because I was growing more and more shy. Restlessly aware of my swollen, mosquito-bitten nose, scraggly beard, lumpy hands. I may have smelled bad, too. They were creamy and spotless. I guess they were disappointed to find the island inhabited.

That was the bad thing about breaking solitude—it made me conscious of my effect. I remembered that I had a personality. It had become unnecessary in just four days. I would have had a more perfect solo if I'd resisted the temptation to talk. But this imperfection was good by way of affording a contrast.

The dominant feature of the play of consciousness while alone was the passivity and receptivity. I've spent lots of time idly wondering about this or that, but it has usually been along the lines already laid down by my education. Being marooned is a bit of a jolt. Being caught in a natural rhythm is, too. The spare diet is another clarifying factor. The total effect is comparable to the mental states of praying, smoking grass, and running/swimming/rowing a long way. Praying—more like Eastern than Western in that Eastern prayer (I'm told) is more incantatory than supplicatory (Lord, hear our prayer), or even contractually demanding (*In te, Domine, speravi: non confundar in aeternum*) as in the Western Church. You aren't actively seeking grace; you're just waiting to see if you're not somehow near it.

Pot—the same occasional rising bubbles of hilarity and clarity. But smoking is much further into introversion. It seems to me that what narrowly increased sensual clarities there are while smoking are paid for by decreased general awareness. At worst, you get nailed down; at best, your trip is on rails. I know a guy who once felt he was the mercury in a thermometer. It was all right, he said, but very . . . specialized.

Running/swimming/rowing can get you into a similar overturning of your usual set of concentrations. But being still on a small island happens idly. Drop by drop, until you brim over. The rhythms of running, et cetera, inevitably become throbbing magnifications of feeling that just as inevitably become various kinds of pain, and that's a different pleasure altogether.

Of course the solo can be unfortunate. Desperately uncomfortable. Freezing and rainy. Boring. I was lucky most of the time. But I thought there were very few people who could fail to be lucky on these apparently barren, actually lush, little islands. I didn't see the possible bad edges of the experience until later. (See the epilogue in this chapter.)

Our watch was surprisingly glad to be reunited on the deck of the pickup ship. José was most candid and exuberant. "I didn't think I'd ever look forward to seeing all your shiny pink faces, man. I really didn't." *Abrazos,* pumping handshakes, thumping on the back. I was glad to see him.

An odd thing happened then. Through a series of coincidences too unlikely to describe, there was on the forward deck a visitor who had smuggled a peanut-butter sandwich in her handbag for George, Slocum watch's psychologist-in-residence. He went forward and was passed this contraband (an hour or so before our welcome-home meal) near the bow. He was forty to fifty feet away from the rest of us castaways. The wheelhouse amidships cut off our view. But the minute George covertly unwrapped the wax paper our nostrils flared. Those of us on the rear deck practically pointed like bird dogs.

"Hey, peanut butter."

"Someone's got some peanut butter."

"Yeah, peanut butter."

A piece of that peanut-butter smell had floated into my nostrils and lit on my brain like a spark on a hearthrug. Three of us as keen as hound dogs. It wasn't that any of us *wanted* George's peanut butter—it was that we were so astonishingly *aware* of it.

We were scraggly, funky, grimy—but our senses were clean.

When we were sitting around that night, José said he'd had a pretty good solo until the last day. He'd noticed that the patrol boat came by every day shortly after noon to check his flags (as a precautionary measure, you tie a different-colored little flag to a prominent tree each day so that the patrol boat can see from afar you're okay). José, therefore, concluded that he would be picked up shortly after noon on the fourth day. In fact, the pickup ship didn't get to his island until evening. He'd been enraged. Most of us had had something of the same expectation and something of the same impatience. Once we'd begun to think about getting back, every minute became galling. We'd all assumed that there was an obligation to pick us up at a certain hour. I can't remember how I'd settled on my probable hour of delivery, but I'd picked one, and I'd been irritated. We all said we wouldn't have minded spending more time, even a couple more days, on our islands, but we felt we'd been made fools of—sitting a half-day on the very spot where we'd been dropped. We felt we had to be right there when the whaler zipped ashore from the pickup ship, but we also felt that since we *were* sitting there, the boat had to show up.

José, whose anxious, irrational period had been longest, compared it to the hassle of appearing in court (presumably on behalf of the organization he worked for, the Real Great

Society). He said he'd finally accepted the waiting outside of courtrooms; it seemed to him the delays were deliberately planned to upset him, and so he fought to keep cool, to win by outwaiting. But he said he'd nearly gone berserk waiting for the pickup, because he'd developed a trust in the competence and benevolence of the Outward Bound people, and he felt betrayed. I got the message: "Now you all know what dependence on 'good people' can be. Worse than messing with bad people."

Jed then made the following points. As it happened, the pickups were all late because of an unintentional snafu. But, he went on, he thought it was a good part of the exercise to upset our dependence on other people's abilities and on the "structure" of the solo. (In fact, in the pre-solo briefing, some staff member had said that we shouldn't be surprised if the pickups were as much as a day late. For some reason we'd all erased that from our thoughts.) Jed said it was a good thing for us to wonder what it would be like to be on our islands indefinitely.

I thought that was okay at the time. Now I can see that this sort of "planning the unplanned" or "unstructuring the structured" is one of the most difficult problems for the staff. The problem is this: Being marooned on an island is, after all, a game. If we really had been shipwrecked or lost, the point of the exercise would be different. We would have spent our time not in meditation but in getting off the damn island. Maybe even building a raft and floating into a shipping channel and flagging down a boat. Or paddling to another inhabited island and bothering some poor fellow on vacation. In short, we'd have upset trade and tourism from Rockland to Castine. In order to have the goodwill of the Coast Guard and the Maine residents, the school does solve problems—it is ready to send a rescue ship, a doctor, or a firefighting team to any of the islands or to the mainland. But in order to challenge its students, the school has to create more problems than it solves, without these problems getting out of control and spilling over into the larger community. The game is stacked against the school. If a student was to raft out and pull a lobster pot—which he would do if he was really afraid of starving—the indignation on the part of the lobsterman would far outweigh any help the school had given hung-up lobster boats. (Yes, Virginia, lobstermen do run aground.) If a student thought he really was abandoned and beavered down some healthy trees to make a raft, the island owner's conservationist indignation would cause him to deny the use of the island to the school. And if too many Outward Bound whaleboats had to be saved by the Coast Guard, the Coast Guard could very well close down the school, since it is, technically, a corporation licensed to carry passengers for hire. It is odd to reflect, while pulling on an oar, that you are legally in the same class as a pleasure-cruise passenger being served a daiquiri under an awning. But on the other hand, if the school ordered the boats in every time the wind blew more than twenty-five knots, the students who had keyed themselves up for high adventure would quite rightly think they might just as well have rented a rowboat in Central Park.

So you can see the thin line the school tightropes between too much artificiality and too much reality. By and large the students *are* challenged and do have adventure. They do have the sensation of being left to their own devices in precarious positions. I don't think anyone has ever breezed through the physical aspects of the course or has felt that he was always safe. Some students have felt occasionally reined in. But some students have given up. They've been hung up on ordinary exercises. They've hitched rides on boats to get off their solo islands, claimed they were sick, balked at the ropes course, the cliff, drownproofing, running up or down the trails around the island, or jumping off the stone wall into the sea. Some have flung their arms around a thwart in the whaleboat as it heeled over in a fresh breeze. So it's very hard for the school to tailor its "challenges" to the different students and stay out of trouble with the neighborhood, the Coast Guard school, benefactors, and parents. However, there are two factors that help the school. They both arise from a change in attitude in the students themselves. I myself came to see by the end that the most dramatic adventures were not the ones geared to the technically competent but those undertaken by the technically incompetent. I think most of the students finally see this and don't clamor for challenges to their particular skills but become interested in challenges to their weak side.

The most extraordinary example of an adventurous incompetence I heard of was in the case of the fifty-yard underwater swim. In the crew doing the exercise there was a boy who couldn't swim at all. He was excused. He stood by, watching his watchmates swim the length of the pond underwater, guided through the dark by a white rope stretched along the bottom. When they had all done it, the nonswimmer said he was going to do it. His instructor tried to dissuade him. He insisted. The instructor agreed he could try, and stationed the rest of the crew along the route. The student jumped in, sank to the bottom (quite a way down), and pulled himself hand over hand along the rope for fifty yards. When he got to the end, the crew on hand pulled him up from the bottom.

I think there are two interesting decisions involved in that story. One is that of the nonswimmer. The other is that of the instructor. The boy had astonishing grit and curiosity. The instructor (and the crew) were willing to go to some trouble and assume some responsibility to give the boy a chance to test himself.

The Hurricane Island school, incidentally, recently gave up this exercise. They feared that a number of students would keep going until they blacked out. The school didn't want to face on a recurring basis the difficulty of getting an unconscious person up from deep water. They also consulted doctors, who gave the school the impression that any blackout, even a short one, might do some harm.

Actually quite a few Outward Bound students are "up for the game," and undertake things they ordinarily wouldn't. It's not from pressure from the school or from the group. Curiosity and grit arose in each person, and the instructors and (more important) the other members of the watch were willing to stand by to help or to take the position that physical accomplishing of any particular feat was not all that important, that an intelligent appraisal of one's physical inability to make an underwater swim, or a climb, or a part of the ropes course was more commendable than making a doomed, frantic attempt that would only demoralize oneself and the rest of the watch.

I'm not saying that this ideal sensitivity existed all the time—just that as a group we tended toward it more and more. I found myself concerned with others' efforts—in fact, gratified by the successes of some guys I wasn't very fond of. A lot of people came to feel this way.

So these two factors—(1) one's realization that the most interesting part of the school does not lie in testing the peripheries of one's technical competence or main strength (both of which nevertheless increase) and (2) one's growing concern for the developing story lines of one's shipmates—help keep the hotbloods from breaking loose.

Another curious development is that the school at first has

an authority that most students accept out of habit, but gradually that staff authority shrinks—"withers away." There is a transfer of reliance on the instructors to reliance on elected captains, then on oneself, and finally on the crew as a whole. There were some rather touching relationships that arose among people in the regular watches and some of the people in our "senior" watch. The youngest boy became a buddy of José's. In fact, José was a glamorous and reassuring figure for a number of the younger boys who were having difficulties. They'd often drop by our tent, not admitting they were looking for José. One evening I was alone in the tent, and Paul dropped in.

Paul: (disappointed) You all alone, huh?

Me: Yeah. You looking for José?

Paul: Nah. I just wanted to see where you guys keep your Geritol. Ha!

Me: José's down at the pier, fishing.

Paul: Fishing. That's a laugh. I'd better go down and show him how. Before he falls in, ha, ha.

These friendships of José's had a lot of side benefits. For one thing, they had a generally warming effect on our whole crew's relationship to the other crews. As a group we might have been aloofly content with one another and our skills. José (along with George) made us more approachable as a whole. For another thing, it was reassuring to some of our crew to realize that these flashes of warmth of José's were the other side of his sometimes alarming flashes of temper.

José was incidentally having other reflections of his own. He said to me once, after a particularly hard day in the boat, "You know, man, I've been talking to these kids from the suburbs. I ask them, 'How come you're always putting out? How come you keep on going with all this?' And they say—now, dig this—they say, 'I dunno.' And that's what it really is, you dig? Maybe that's what some of my people need."

I disagreed that blind endurance was a desirable quality. He said he didn't mean to make it blind—just add that doggedness to get further and faster. He thought that what his people (both blacks and Puerto Ricans) wanted was often more interesting and attractive than what the suburban white kids wanted, but he dug the way the suburban program kept even the tail end of the group moving.

It is true—as José saw—that a lot of the kids there keep trying at first just because someone has set up goals for them. Show most middle-class American kids a program and they'll embrace it. And once they've taken step one, they won't quit. That may be a useful quality, but the sad thing is, a lot of people end up having more feeling for the program—completing the program—than they do for anything else: the other people, the discoveries they make, the new urges that are unearthed. Programs can have a dreary side; they can have the effect of making people dig in just to get certified. Examples: Ph.D. candidates who find themselves slaving for the Ph.D. as the goal rather than the incident of their work. Big-game trophy hunters whose vision narrows to such a point that they see the record clearer than the animal.

Now, a fair number set out in Outward Bound to get certified as salty adventurers. I include myself. I never quite lost that feeling, but I found my peripheral vision widening. I think this happened to a lot of the certification seekers. I'm not sure how much of this was personally inevitable and how much was engineered by subtle pedagogy, but toward the end of the program, the goals became less a matter of performing an activity in a specified manner and more a matter of rising spirits.

•◆•

WHAT COUNTRY, FRIENDS, IS THIS?

By the time we left for final expedition we were aspiring to be at sea. Even—to some extent—with one another. Earlier we might have been determined to move the boat in spite of everything (me, him, you, the rest of them).

We didn't take Jed or Perry on our final expedition. We elected a captain, first mate, and quartermaster (a key job, that—doling out food). As it happened, the captain and the first mate (the two alleged sailors—Don and me) were among the few who were at any time actively seasick. Our first problem was not getting too far ahead of the convoy. Staying in convoy—five whaleboats—was difficult psychologically and physically. The convoy idea came as rather a surprise. We thought it was an impeding detail sprung somewhat late in the course. It was frustrating, because our crew was rather proud of the way we'd learned to move our boat—with fair speed, pretty well on course, and with accommodation to one another.

The first day we had a fresh breeze for a while. We'd get out in front, heave to while the other boats caught up, and then run like hell to keep from getting rammed as the other boats bore down on us, wildly out of control.

For lunch we tore apart a fatty canned ham with our rigging knives and fingers. We found some cheese for José, who didn't like pig meat. We discovered that navigating—like reading in a car—made our then navigator queasy. The wind moved into the southeast, and a cold fog rolled in on top of a greasy ground swell. We were informed by the staff whaleboat that we were supposed to follow the appointed lead boat, which was MacMillan watch. We did. We all got lost. The wind died, although the ground swell kept bobbing us around.

We rowed around for a while, conferring with MacMillan watch as to where we were, and, more important, where we might spend the night. We decided to backtrack toward Brimstone Island, embarrassingly close to home. The fog grew thicker, but we finally spotted a piece of island between fogbanks. We collectively and mistakenly identified it and altered course. After another hour we found another piece of island and some rocks, which caused some navigational surprise. But these pieces of the jigsaw puzzle weren't at all ambiguous, and we figured out where we were for certain. Off into the fog again, and after an even colder hour, MacMillan found Brimstone. It was treeless, forebodingly ringed by rocks, and rocky itself. Fortunately, someone had spent his solo there and guided us around to a pebbly beach.

The staff whaleboat rowed away to spend their night in (we suspected) a nicer spot.

After an hour of hating the place as I gathered firewood, I suddenly found myself falling for it. Above the steep rocky shore there was a plateau—a series of small meadows. My duffelmate (John Tingley) and I set up a remarkably comfortable shelter in an open nook of rock that gave us two natural walls and a grass bed. The fog grew thicker, but it didn't grow colder. We could just make out the spot below us by the glow of four tiny fires and by the muffled sound of fortysome people crunching through the pebbles.

Woke up at ten that night to go on anchor watch. My partner was from another watch. He was about eighteen, I guessed. We sat on the beach, ready to rouse the men sleeping on the island if the anchors broke loose. We couldn't see the boats in the fog, but we could check by feel the tightening and slacking of the lines to shore. As each swell came in, the lines from stern to shore went limp. As the water receded and the boats were pulled away, the shorelines grew taut. In fact, they lifted off the beach and practically hummed.

As the two of us sat there, we got involved in a strangely discontinuous conversation, because whoever wasn't talking was awake for only every other word. I was talking about how Orwell really began to believe in the ideally humane side of socialism (fraternity—the common decency of most people) only after he'd served in the ranks in a militia in the Spanish Civil War, an experience that for some reason then struck me as similar to Outward Bound. Except no one was shooting at us. A rather large exception, but I pressed on. My companion was talking about how sad it was that the people in his watch (MacMillan) had become frozen into roles. Group leader role. Just-one-of-the-guys role. Sad sack. How the role-playing had been a great disappointment to him. Especially, I gathered, as he had a lousy role. I missed some of this. Then there came a moment when our conversations intersected. Something about rites of initiation—the lack of them in our culture. But suddenly, with the careful, embarrassed solicitude of a young man for an older man, he said I looked really tired and asked me if I didn't want to take a nap. He said he'd watch the anchor lines by himself, and if he got tired he'd wake me up. I said I had more to say, but my next waking moment was at midnight when our relief came. My co-watcher pointed me up the hill to my shelter, and politely added that he'd liked our talk.

The fog was breaking up the next morning, but slowly, since there was no wind. I toured the island with some others. We were amazed to find an untended flock of sheep in the uppermost meadow.

We had pleasant rowing all morning. A light breeze came up by lunchtime, and we suddenly had a sparkling blue September afternoon. I went on bow watch and was able to strip down and dry my socks and long underwear on a mainstay. It was a great pleasure to know where we were. Plentiful nuns and cans through Merchants Row and up Blue Hill Bay. We decided to go on when the first stars came out. It was still dusky light. The wind began to die. We went on under both sails and oars. Still very blithe.

Then, abruptly, complete darkness. One of the rowers in another boat got stomach cramps. His captain hailed the staff boat, which in turn hailed us to heave to while they investigated. We couldn't keep our kerosene running lights lit to warn off other boats. Two boats collided in the dark. We paddled about, trying to keep in touch but trying also to stay clear as the other boats' sails caught puffs of wind and pushed them about in the dark. The tide was by now set against us, and we were still short of our campsite. The boy with cramps didn't seem too badly off, so we tried rowing on, but there was no way of measuring if we were making any progress at all. We couldn't use our sails, we decided, because we had to stay only a boat's length apart to see one another, and the puffs of wind were likely to jam us together with some force. In the previous collision no one had been hurt, but there had been a few bruises from the oar butts swinging out of control. Still, we were for pressing on. The staff boat overruled us. They also had no idea where we were, so they wanted us to stay put. We poked in toward a long island that was supposed to be to the east of us, but we couldn't be sure where the rocks were. Finally, after narrowly missing some submerged crags while trying to lead us into land, the staff boat announced we would spend the night in the boats. We rafted the boats in pairs and set our anchors. There was a strong tide running. One of the school lobster boats, called in by radio, showed up in case the boy with cramps had to be unloaded. The doctor decided he was okay. Mr. Root, from the staff boat, borrowed the lobster boat's dinghy to go around checking up on how well we were rafted and anchored. I was sitting on my rowing thwart, drowsing off against the gunwale, when Mr. Root boarded us. I dimly remember him handing me the painter of the dinghy. A few moments passed. I heard a voice saying, "Mr. Root, you planning to spend the night with us?" I recognized that that question had something to do with me, but I couldn't pin it down.

Clamor. Consternation. I woke up all the way. The dinghy was disappearing on the tide at a rapid pace. It was only a boat's length off our rafted sterns, but we were at anchor. We uncleated our anchor lines and paid them out as both boats backwatered to catch the dinghy. It was just out of reach as we came to the end of our anchor lines. It disappeared into the fog.

Mr. Root hailed the staff boat and cursed me. Mr. Root hailed the lobster boat and cursed me. Mr. Root sounded the alarm on our Freon horn and cursed me, but he'd begun to repeat himself.

We all sat in chilled silence for ten minutes while the lobster boat chugged downstream cautiously. It had a depth indicator, but it drew several feet of water, and we were in close to shoals. It looked as though the dinghy was gone. Mr. Root cleared his throat and asked me why I hadn't jumped in and swum for it.

I had, in fact, considered it, even though the water was forty or so. It wasn't much above that in the air. A particle of common sense allowed me to see that that was a ridiculous idea. But I was cast down. I'd been determined to become an impeccable salt while in Maine.

The lobster boat finally caught up with its dinghy and came back to relieve us of Mr. Root. We settled down for the night. Some of the adjoining crew thought I'd let go of the boat on purpose and that it was a neat way of paying back the authority that had condemned us to a night on the water. I felt the least I could do was take the least desirable watch (we had to maintain a watch in this case, for fear that a cruising boat would bear down on us in the fog). It was very cold. We all shivered, but some managed to sleep. When I went off watch (at about two a.m.), I informed the other boat that it was their turn to post a man. The Pollard first mate had already stood watch himself, and he was anxious to rouse someone. He couldn't. He shook people. He kicked people. No one got up. The acting captain got up, woken by the noise. He said he'd take watch, but the first mate said no and ended up taking the watch himself. I stayed up to talk with him for a while. He told me how things stood with his crew.

Their elected captain had turned out really not to care for the expedition at all. By default, almost all the sailing, steering, and navigating were done by a guy named Oscar, who became the acting captain. Paul (the quartermaster) and Vince (the first mate) helped him out, but almost everyone else was caught in the downward spiral of ill feeling and despondency. Both Paul and Vince were angry, and only grudgingly did more than their share. Vince's rage in particular drove the sluggards into deeper resentful sluggishness. Oscar was the iron man. He'd been either at the tiller or rowing from five-thirty in the morning until nine-thirty at night. Sixteen hours. He also did the navigating. Vince's rage wasn't just on his own behalf but on behalf of Oscar, about whom he'd come to feel protective. His admiration, I think, widened the gap between the few doers and the non-doers. Vince would say, "Look at him, you bastards, he's doing all your work," and the non-doers would say, "Yeah. Look at him."

The fog was as thick as ever at dawn. Dead calm. Pollard was the lead boat that day, and we were treated to the sight of Oscar and Vince rousing the necessary oarsmen. There was a carrot as well as the stick that Vince provided, a couple of swift kicks with his seaboot. The carrot was that we had to get to a beach of some kind before we could have a hot breakfast. We'd skipped supper the night before. Also, we were all so stiff and cold that rowing was the only way to get warm.

Oscar led us toward the island, checked out the size and height, and decided where we were. He led us on through the fog to a can. He was twenty yards off after a mile or so of rowing. Just near enough to see it. He hit the next can dead-on, which was remarkable. The Pollard rowers were spent by the time we got to a beach. It wasn't just a question of physical fatigue—it was a question of downheartedness. There wasn't the least bit of buoyancy in them. They barely talked to one another. In fact, they barely took an interest in anything but being individually miserable. I'd never had much faith in the concept of *morale* before. I'd thought—about football or soccer or moving furniture—that if something went wrong, you either weren't strong enough or weren't smart enough. You weren't up to the job, period, no more explanations. But these guys were up to the job, as they showed later. But at that moment they were so demoralized that even a skeptic like me could *see* it.

We had a long, big, hot breakfast on the beach in Fogg Cove. Sausages, applesauce, chicken stew (from last night's non-supper), oatmeal, and tea. Mr. Root and I convened over tea and some leftover staff stew. Mutual apologies. I'd always been fond of Mr. Root, who was normally very loose. Had it been anyone other than Mr. Root swearing at me the night before, my embarrassment would have turned to anger. In fact, had it been one of the two wiseasses in the staff boat, I would have taken a poke at him, and one of us would have gone swimming for the dinghy. As it was, Mr. Root and I got to be buddies.

We set off again, beginning our circumnavigation of Mount Desert Island. Fairly soon the usual midday southwesterly caught up with us, and we were doing well under sail. The wind got stiffer and stiffer. By the time we got to the narrows at the northern tip (a big island—it has a national park, a couple of good mountains, and the only real fjord on our seacoast), the wind was mixed with rain and blowing good and hard. We waited around all hove-to while the lead boat and the staff boat dickered about how much water there was in the channel, the state of the tide, and the softness of the bottom. We got madder and madder. Our good wind was blowing on by while we sat in the rain. Nadir of staff-boat popularity. We'd been told that the expedition was entirely in our hands, and here it clearly wasn't. We had to dump our mizzens and reef our mainsails. We crawled through the narrows after more than an hour of waiting. We thought there were better ways of proceeding.

During the afternoon we sailed down Frenchman Bay to Burnt Porcupine Island, northeast of Bar Harbor. We landed in the dark. Tingley and I erected the second (and, as it turned out, the last) of our sumptuous shelters. We awarded ourselves our second Frank Lloyd Wright medal of excellence for the use of plastic, rock, and grass. We then fell into pits of deep, dark sleep.

The next day started late and never ended. We were trying to sail into the teeth of a sharp wind that kept shifting every time we tacked. The wind was supposed to be from the southwest. In theory we all should have been able to sail either south or west. With the sprit rigs we were using we really couldn't count on anything better, but we couldn't even do that. When we headed south, the wind came out of the south, and when we headed west, the wind came out of the west. By lunchtime we'd made almost no progress, although we'd sailed a long way back and forth across the bay. We broke out the oars and rowed into the wind and into some good-sized waves that were rolling up the bay, frequently whitecapped.

As we were bobbing around, waiting for the other boats to catch up, I suddenly found myself clutching my oar. Violent seasickness.

By late afternoon the staff boat suggested a halt. We unanimously rejected that idea and won out. By suppertime a fog came up. Onward. We knew where we were. There was an element of rage in our attitude now. Darkness and more fog. The staff boat expressed concern as we'd made the turn around Cadillac Mountain (which we never saw), and Mount Desert Island was now a lee shore. The wind had shifted to the southeast, which meant that we could sail, but it also meant more fog and cold coming in from the whole reach of the Atlantic. Our captain was now sick. I crawled back from bow watch. Tingley put me to the recovery test: He said, "How'd you like a caramelled apple?" I passed. Barely.

The staff boat had earlier been trying to signal us for some reason. Our then helmsman thought they were telling us we

were far enough south to make the turn around the bottom
of Mount Desert Island. In fact, they were just up to their
old tricks, wanting to pull into the nearest cove for another
night in the boats. It began to rain in earnest. Because of our
premature turn we were no longer exactly sure where we were.
We sailed on. The staff boat blew their horn for a rendezvous.
We were worn out and cold but still wanted to press on. The
staff boat was afraid we were in for a bad storm. The wind had
picked up considerably. We could hear the surf to the north.
We maintained that we knew—give or take a half-mile—
where we were. The staff boat—quite rightly—wasn't willing to give or take a half-mile. Especially since the last boat
in the convoy was having trouble sailing. Not their fault—
something was wrong with their centerboard.

We were disarmed by the staff's allurements. They shouted
to us that perhaps we could get ashore if we'd trust them. We
all dumped our sails and moved nose-to-tail into a cove. Of
course, once we were there it turned out that there was not
much shelter from the sea. It was also clear from the noise of
the surf that the seas were running too high to make a landing
in the dark. And again, although we knew which cove we were
in, it was uncertain where the rocks were.

We rafted up with Pollard again and dropped anchors. It
was about ten o'clock and the coldest night so far. It was now
pelting rain. We pulled the mainsail out of its bag and bun-
dled together in a body pod for warmth. The heap of bodies in foul-weather gear looked like a jarful of bright yellow
worms. Mike—our six-foot-four seminarian—stretched from
gunwale to gunwale, his long shanks draped over the centerboard trunk. We laid the oars across the thwarts to make a
platform. We couldn't put anyone in the bilge, where there
was now six inches of water, a combination of leakage, rain,

and spray. I had worked out a comfortable position. No, not comfortable, but better than standing out in the rain. Unfortunately, I discovered, among other symptoms of discomfort, that I had to piss. Of all times. I unlocked my elbows and feet from the body pod and squirmed out from under the sail. We were tossing quite a lot, and our rafting lines had loosened so that every third wave or so we bumped gunwales with Pollard. Kneeling and leaning over the gunwales (but not pissing to windward), I nearly went over the side after a hard bump. I was afraid that we would do some serious damage, but I couldn't tighten the rafting lines. I sat for a while, fending off Pollard's gunwale with my feet. I was afraid I'd be stuck with the job. I tried again to tighten the lines. I was about to give up when Mr. Root appeared in a dinghy. The school lobster boat had traced us with its radar and followed us into the cove. Mr. Root was pleased to find someone on watch—a complete accident of my having to take a leak. He had a partial solution to the problem. We rigged spring lines—our stern to their bow, their stern to our bow. This arrangement took the strain off the stern-to-stern and bow-to-bow lines, and we were able to tighten them. And thus, in turn, to tighten the spring lines, and so forth. We got the boats back together and some fenders in place. The Pollard first mate and our seasick captain dragged themselves out to help.

It was clear that the wind and sea were not abating. We had to post a watch, both to tighten the lines periodically and to make sure we weren't dragging our anchor toward the shore, invisible but audible.

I looked at our captain, and he looked at me. He was luminously green in the face, even by the red glow of our running light.

I discovered two things in the next hour (we'd shortened

the watches to one hour, since by then we had only six hours until dawn). One was that no amount of clothing can keep you warm in a wet wind. I had on long fishnet underwear, khaki pants, wool pants, a wool shirt, an Ensolite flotation jacket, and foul-weather gear on top of everything. I've never been colder, even hunting all day in Iowa in below-zero weather. The only close second I could think of was a half hour I'd spent waiting for a bus in Chicago in January. The tears coming out of one eye had frozen it shut. But this was worse. It was above freezing, but the sensation of cold was in my very center. Not just hands, or feet, or face, but deep in my empty stomach. The second thing I discovered was that it was somehow exhilarating. I wasn't making up the excitement. It came in unconscious flashes. Something had slipped into me during the last four days of rowing and sailing. Or perhaps over a longer period. I found that for several seconds at a time I was pleased to be there, on that boat, in that weather. But then I'd huddle in the stern and feel sorry for myself. Then along would come another bubble, and I would feel elated again. *Let's see just how cold I can get and decide not to care.*

I reached the limits of this elation. After my hour was up, I laid hands on Loong-Ho Tan under the sail and asserted that—by the powers vested in me as first mate and in the name of that fairness common to all systems of government and religion—it was his turn to go on watch.

I discovered that I couldn't fit into the space under the sail that Loong-Ho had left. I tucked the sail back in and retired to the stern. I remembered a plastic sheet in the loose mess duffel. The other sheets were lashed around personal gear to keep it dry, and I couldn't find it in myself to expose someone's change of clothes to the rain and spray. I found the one sheet and wrapped myself in it. It went round me, head to toe, three times. I lay on the helmsman's thwart. I found that the plastic gave support to the parts of me that hung off the thwart. I fell asleep.

I was woken up by a sharp crackling and splintering noise. I was sure the boat was aground. I couldn't get out of the sheet. I thought I was underwater. My arms were pinned. I couldn't tell which way was up. After a moment of panic I realized it was just Loong-Ho trying to wrap himself into the loose end of the sheet. The stiff plastic around my head was making the noise. Loong-Ho was apologetic. Purely as a bribe to keep him out of the plastic sheet while he was on watch, I gave him my foul-weather jacket. This was later chalked up as a good deed. I have great feeling for Loong-Ho, but this was self-defense.

At four or so I happened to roll off the thwart and wake up. By some miracle of persuasion, someone in the Pollard boat was on watch. I lifted the edge of the sail. Loong-Ho was somehow near the middle of the pile. It may have been a writhing mass of yellow worms, but it was home. I dove in. After a few minutes, I realized it was warm. Not just a little warmer, but positively, comfortably, miraculously warm. Occasionally as I was dozing off, I had an urge to lift the edge of the sail to get a breath of fresh air, but I always decided in favor of lying still.

At four-forty, there was inexplicable mass hysteria. Tingley happened to wake up beside Mike. Tingley asked him what time it was. Mike told him. Tingley for some reason found it both funny and incredible that it was four-forty. "Twenty of *five*? Of *five*? *Before* five? Wait. Not five. Four-*forty*." Other voices joined in to assure Tingley that it was almost five. He denied them all. I don't know why this was funny. Then Tingley asked whose foot was by his ear. No one knew. Tingley asked everyone. It was no one's. That struck us as endlessly funny. We lay there, no one moving but everyone roaring with laughter. As it subsided, George said, "José, can you see by the dawn's early light?" He'd said it before, but it set us off again.

We dozed again, and then at five-fifteen we all woke up together and leapt to our feet. We didn't say anything, but we knew we wanted to get moving. The wind had shifted. It was blowing strong out of the northeast. That was our wind, and we didn't want to miss a puff. Home was to the southwest. Everyone else was roused. No one said a word about stopping for a hot breakfast. We all smelled the stable. We set sail for home, thirty-five to forty miles away. We reached south to get to the channel and then ran before the wind. Even when we altered course slightly, the wind seemed to stay behind us. We practically surfed home. The waves would curl up behind our pointed stern and slither by, giving us a shove. It was like rushing down a fast river in a canoe. It was as though a friendly whale were going our way, scratching his back on the belly of our boat.

It never got warm enough that day so that our feet ever woke up, but we were happy enough.

Some of the guys were wary, however, of hoping. I said out loud that if the wind held, we'd get home by suppertime. Two people said, "Don't say that!"

We knocked off the remains of a gallon of peanut butter and a pound of cheese. We finished off cans of ginger ale that were supposed to be reserved for the seasick. It felt like riotous banqueting. By the time we went past Stonington there was nothing left of the spare rations but bouillon cubes and oatmeal flakes. All the while we were sailing along. For about nine hours. We gauged our average speed at close to four knots, although it dropped off by the end. We were going five at times. By yachting standards that may seem dull, but it was a thrill.

One alarming incident. On Pollard, one of the crew (possibly upset at the division of food) took a swing at little Paul. Paul took a swing back. We heard Paul's voice cut through the wind—"You think cuz you're so damn big you can push me around; well, I'm gonna wrap an oar around your head!" We cheered Paul. Oscar left the helm and mizzen sheet to Vince and sprang forward to separate the two. The staff captain called through his bullhorn, "Hey, Oscar! What do you do in your *spare* time?"

Just as we reached Hurricane Island there was a lull in the wind. We broke out our oars to make the mooring. It was well before supper.

There was a curious stillness about the island. We automatically took care of the boat and gear. We felt for a moment embarrassingly anticlimactic, dazed.

Jed asked us what we thought of our expedition. I later wished I'd thought of Gertrude Stein and said, "When we got there, there was no there there." But that's not true; there was some there there.

A number of us happened to take our boots off simultaneously in our six-man tent with the flaps tied shut. We'd had our boots on for two whole days straight. It was like a gas attack. My own feet were a study in fungus-white and chilblain-purple.

Loong-Ho and Pat and I set out on a run around the island. It was just restlessness. It was an urge to stretch out and assert ourselves on firm land. It was particularly nice to run through the spruce woods. Sweet-smelling and wind-sheltered.

There was no hot water for showers, so we went for a swim in the quarry. Sweet freshwater. I found some dry, clean clothes. A pair of old khakis felt like silk. Dry wool socks. The last bit of numbness left my feet; I could feel every wool fiber as I

scratched around with my toes. Caress of an old sweatshirt. All
the clothes seemed to float on me after the weight of wet wool
and foul-weather gear. Even my work boots felt light. Walking
down to the mess hall, I loved every step. I felt as hollow and
light as a gull and as clean as marble.

This feeling persisted until late that night. I woke up in my
bunk, certain that I was in the boat. We were being driven
onto the rocks. I wandered around the tent, looking for an oar.
I kept from falling overboard by holding on to the cot railings
and the tent pole. I thought it was the mizzenmast. I finally
realized where I was. I climbed back into my sleeping bag and
listened to the wind and the rain with great relief.

This kind of dreaming was a common phenomenon. Pat
woke us up by calling out from his dreamed bow watch,
"Rocks! Rocks! Come to port!" He was kneeling on his bunk
with his head stuck out in the rain. Another guy woke his
tent up by shouting, "She's not coming about! Backwind the
main!" He was standing outside in a puddle, shoving the tent
flap into the wind.

•◆•

Last two days. We spent the next to last chopping down
selected tall spruce as pilings for the pier. It was still raining.
Perry led us through the woods to find the trees. It was Snow
White and twelve dwarfs.

The last full day was supposed to be a day of competitions—
six-mile steeplechase, ropes course, wall and beam, mile rowing race, et cetera. Unfortunately, a hurricane was reported
to be on its way. The school decided to hold the six-mile race

anyway. As usual, we did our pre-breakfast run and jump into the sea. Not the full two and a half miles, however, in view of the six to come.

We lined up for the race an hour after breakfast. Ninety-six of us on the volleyball court. Some of the staff ran, too. We listened to the instructions. First a mile circuit around the middle of the island, including a long gradual hill to thin out the pack. One mile. Then around the outer edge of the island twice. $2 \times 2.5 = 5 + 1 = 6$. It was raining hard. The few flat parts of the run were more than half underwater, held in pools by the roots that crossed the trail. It was hard to guess how deep the water was, and even after you'd been around the course it was hard to remember. The east side of the island was the flat path through the main camp, and then the trail through the spruces, climbing steadily toward the north end. Huge flat angles of wet rock. Slippery going up and slippery going down. Between the mounds of rock the patches of ground were mud wallows. The west side of the island started with a steep downhill from the north end. Then the trail ran along the shore. It was a series of jumps from boulder to boulder. The rocks came to an end with a spectacular long sharp spine known as the Whale's Back. And then a winding trail through a meadow and more woods to the home stretch.

I was nervous beforehand. I hadn't been in a race since I'd run in high school. Tingley, who had run cross-country in high school before taking up swimming in college, remembered the old pre-race sincerity ploy: "I know I'm not going to do well, but gosh, John, I sure hope you do." The earnest jocks—about half of the group—went through warm-up exercises. Jed, who has run the Boston Marathon in less than three hours, told us they didn't make much difference.

When the starting gun went off, a phalanx sprinted out.

Five or six runners were spilled and somewhat trampled. Fortunately, Pat (our watch's hope, along with Tingley) got out front with the other pre-race favorites.

Pat's race was very exciting. He kept trading off the lead with another sinewy runner, who kept trying to push the pace without actually leaving Pat behind. Apparently, getting too far ahead can be upsetting. This is hearsay on my part.

But Pat needed the other guy for different reasons. Pat, who is nearsighted, found that his glasses were too awash with rain for him to be able to pick out his footing coming down from the north end. Both times they were going up the rocks, he feinted the other fellow into the lead and then half blindly followed in his footsteps. The last time around, Pat followed his rival down and passed him in the lower rocks just before the Whale's Back, under a mile out. He was relying as much on memory as on sight. Pat was wary of the other guy's kick, so he pressed hard and built up a lead. In the final mud stretch he was out to a fifty-yard lead, but the second man closed fast. Pat's calves cramped. He hunched over for a few steps, then straightened up and flew. He won by a couple of yards. Forty-four minutes. Considering the scrabbly terrain and the rain, an impressive race. Even the staff was impressed. The first staff runner came in seventh. Most of the top ten runners would be capable of five miles in about thirty minutes in a regular cross-country race—over a golf course, for example.

Tingley came in nineteenth in about forty-eight minutes. I came in thirty-second in fifty-two minutes. Just made the top third of the field. Mike came in a few steps behind me. Tingley, Mike, and I felt we'd done okay for the Geritol watch. Pat, of course, was our hero, radiant in victory. His younger brother had won the race in his Outward Bound course in Colorado.

My chief private pleasure was that I'd kept after it all the way. I also remembered the trail fairly well, and so was able to swoop headlong down some slopes in the woods, knowing there was a tree to grab to help swing me through the turn at the bottom.

Tingley, Mike, and I all beat a college half-miler who had looked fast. Indeed, he was fast, and on the level stretches he would lope by Mike and me, but we'd catch him when we clambered up the rocks. Second lap around the island, we lost him.

I had some afterthoughts. There'd been a clump of four runners fifteen yards in front of me for the last mile. I thought I should have tried to pass them at least a half-mile out. I ran hard at the finish, but not *soon* enough. The five of us finished in a spray of mud, a lot of which I swallowed. The afterthought didn't hold. I'd thudded across the finish on peg legs and stayed on my feet only because Tingley caught me. He put his spare wool shirt around me. Later, when I tried to give it back, he said, "No. Keep it. Good-luck shirt. You'll be racing again."

There was a lot of this exuberance and goodwill, which was just as well, since the rain was driving in at more of a slant as we caught some of the hurricane. We all spent the rest of the day hauling boats out of the water. The peapods, the Boston Whalers, the small sailboats. The whaleboats were towed off in strings by the lobster boats to a creek some miles away. We'd stripped them of gear and rigging so they could be sunk in the creek to save them from the storm. We worked hard all day, still caught up in the semi-emergency, semi-festival atmosphere.

We dumped all the tents. When we got to Jed and Perry's and lowered the canvas in a heap over their cots and bookshelf, Perry said, "I told you to pay the rent, Paw."

Once we had the boats and the island ready for the storm, it didn't come. We caught some gusts of wind and rain, but the center looped off to sea at the last minute. It was like the hurricane in *Rise and Fall of the City of Mahagonny*. "The hurricane has around the city of Mahagonny a detour gemacht! / O wonderful rescue!"

We met for our farewell supper at two a.m. and cheered at the news that the Rockland ferry would show up after all. We wrote a page or two apiece of impressions and suggestions for the school's records ("The hurricane was just right. Be sure to have one next time."). Without a drop of liquor, we were reeling around in full banquet style. Then, after each watch officer talked to his crew, we lined up to receive our badges for the course. A number of students said they couldn't accept the badges because they'd broken the pledge we'd taken in the beginning. They'd either smoked or got hold of some booze or—and this was a reason for some—they felt they had not "lived in good fellowship." Not much was made of this at all, but I was struck by it. Imagine the resoluteness of the first person to say no. After he spoke up there was a moment of quietness in the dining hall. It was the end of a twenty-one-hour day as well as the end of the course. There were more than a hundred of us, including staff. For this guy, age eighteen, the past month was possibly the most prolonged intense experience of his life. And he stood up and said no, he can't take a badge, he feels that at some point he broke his pledge.

I knew some of the guys who turned down their badges. I think they wanted their badges, but they had come to want the month they'd had even more—just as it was. I got the impression that this was a spontaneous and personal, not an imposed, scrupulousness.

We'd turned in all of the Outward Bound gear except for

our sleeping bags. We sacked out on the floor of the machine shop in the boathouse for the few hours before dawn. I went for a walk. I was tempted to pull out my pipe and a bit of tobacco I'd kept in my ditty bag. Technically I was de-pledged, and I was in a very reflective mood now that the wind had died and the stars were out. But I began to drowse on my feet. I found a spot on the boathouse floor, and I had that curious sensation of being able to dive down to the bottom of sleep.

. ➤ .

EPILOGUE

During the last few days at Hurricane Island, I'd begun to think of it as a combination of Delphi and Olympia. Delphi: jagged rock and evergreen, a place of pilgrimage whose oracle more often than not told you to work it out for yourself. Olympia: a gathering of amateur athletes in a setting of natural beauty—soft mounds of surrounding hills that seem to hold the center of the earth. The landscape must have made both triumph and defeat less jarring, and I imagine that the effect of Olympia must have been to make the events themselves seem as much a celebration as winning.

The day we all left I'd had two conversations that put me onto the darker side. On the dock waiting for the ferry, I fell into conversation with my co-watcher from Brimstone Island. It was a sparkling fall day. We were both a little cold. Suddenly we were talking about how he thought he'd failed. He'd been trying to discover whether he was a coward or not, and he'd concluded that he was. That he was afraid perhaps of physical violence, perhaps of confrontation, perhaps of fear itself. I'd known he'd been pushed around by some of the members of his watch, but I hadn't thought it had gone very far. I knew the captain and the first mate, and was sure they would have stepped in. But, he now told me, he was curious about his inability to fight, and so he'd kept on deliberately provoking his chief antagonists. Each time he'd get knocked around. But he never got sufficiently angry enough to throw a punch himself. So he was sure he was inadequate, but he'd kept heading back into the storm, trying to *observe* the precise moment of weakness (as he thought) in himself.

For a half hour we discussed the nature of cowardice and violence. He was afraid that this reluctance of his meant that he didn't have a "grasp on reality." I said that that didn't follow, and from what I'd seen and from what he'd told me it was clear that he wasn't a coward, and that what he counted as inadequacy and missing reality may have been a greater sensitivity to reality. I argued that he hadn't tested himself fairly, since the very fact of his self-observation put him at a disadvantage, might have puzzled people, and people who are puzzled get pissed off. And so on. I don't think he found any comfort in these ideas, but he weighed them. He wasn't looking for comfort. He paused and then said, "I've watched you here."

"Oh."

"I think you have some of the same problems I do. No. Not the same but something . . . There's a way of being right that makes people mad." He paused. "But you got along. Your group got along. You liked each other. They liked you."

"After I fell off the cliff."

"Maybe that's it. You can be funny. I'm not funny. I fell off, too." He looked at me hard. "Did you fall on purpose?"

"I'm not *that* funny."

He said, "Maybe things get better just by getting older."

"Yes."

"But you can't say why."

"Not easily. But they do. I'm sorry. I'm not much help."

He said he thought he could work out the answer himself now that he had some reason to think there was an answer. He may have meant that, or he may have been politely ending the conversation. We separated to join our watches for group snapshots.

I was shaken by his harsh experimentation on himself. By his judgment of himself. By how little he valued the curiosity and nerve it took to keep on with his experiment.

My wife met me on the dock in Rockland. I came ashore with Pat, José, and John Tingley, who all charmed her. They boarded the bus for Boston while my wife and I drove off for a second breakfast. We were on the highway somewhere near Portland when we picked up a hitchhiker. He was from Out-ward Bound. He'd been left in the men's room at a rest stop when the bus left.

By then I'd told most of the story to my wife, who believed the physical side ("You're thin, all right") but was skeptical of the psychological side. Our hitchhiker climbed in, and after thirty seconds of recognition of me and introduction to my wife, he suddenly opened his heart to her. He talked practically nonstop from Portland to Boston. He confirmed—enlarged on—what I'd just been saying. He was an English boy. Or per-haps Welsh. He was now living in Canada. Something trig-gered him—perhaps my wife's interest, perhaps relief that he was going to catch his plane after all. He was the most volatile talker I'd heard in a long time. He really felt that he had discovered a truth about all mankind and his relation to it. He felt he'd learned how to behave decently. With honor. "Not that I *did* act well. I didn't see it till the end. Perhaps I wouldn't have seen it except for Mr. Lee." Mr. Lee was his watch officer. Praise of Mr. Lee for several minutes. Then, "No, I must have seen it in any case. I behaved quite badly at first. I mean, we had several rotten fellows in our watch. Complete swine, really. No thought for others. Pigged the rations in the boat. It made us all behave badly. Then we began to understand, to see what one must do, how one must behave. It was marvelous at the end, don't you think? The way everything collapsed. The tents. And the authority. But not into chaos. Not even some of our tough lot." It was true—objectively—that he'd been in the most difficult watch. One of them had run off with a school motorboat, which was recovered near Rockland. It apparently hadn't occurred to the guy to *say* he wanted to leave, which is the much easier way of getting to the mainland. But then he may have been avoiding going back where he'd come from, whether it was home or a reform school. Another guy, resenting the others' telling him to clean up the tent, crapped on the rock that served as a front stoop. Our hitchhiker thought that even the tough guys had changed some, and that, more important, he had come to sympathize with them. He had turned down his badge, however, because he thought he failed to "live in good fellowship" as well as he could have. Still, he felt he'd learned enough to revise his life. I thought I'd just met two characters from Russian novels—the first from Dostoyevsky, the second from Tolstoy.

I don't know how long the drive took. Probably a couple of hours. We were sorry to see him go. He loped off into the airport. Slightly gangly, dressed in baggy clothes still stiff with dried salt. A floppy hat, steel-rimmed glasses, and a few whiskers. Under one arm his knapsack and half a loaf of bread (we hadn't had time to stop at a restaurant, but since he hadn't eaten since dawn, we stopped at a grocery store). After a minute he jogged back to say he was in fact in time for the plane. He thanked us and loped off again into the crowd, oblivious of the people staring at him. I felt I should get out and explain to them where he'd come from, what he'd just done, who he was.

·◆·

TWO DOGS

A couple of months later, in mid-November, I was still mulling over Outward Bound. My feelings had been hurt. I'd asked my watch officer, whom I admired a lot, whether I could get a job as an assistant watch officer. He said no—I was too impatient with people who weren't already eager and competent. I wondered whether that was true or not. And if it was, whether I minded.

One afternoon, I set out for a long walk with our two dogs. We'd come ashore for the winter, since Narragansett Bay sometimes froze. We were temporarily living in a stone house among some wooded hills south of the Great Swamp in Rhode Island. I left the path for some reason—curiosity, mostly. The basset got far ahead of me and began to yelp that she was lost or stuck. I went after her. The Labrador and I caught up with her in a rhododendron grove. I made both dogs heel and went back toward the trail, which was just over a ridge I'd come down. The trail wasn't there. I crashed around and ended up by a small pond. A fog had blown in. I crashed around some more. It was suddenly dark. I tried going back to the rhododendron grove. I banged my shins. I knocked down buckets of water from the wet leaves. I tore my pants leg. I kept thrashing, resisting having to admit I was lost. After a long time, I was exhausted and baffled. I couldn't have started getting lost more than two miles from the house, and certainly not more than a couple of hundred yards from the trail. But I had no idea which way I had stampeded myself. Or how far.

I climbed a tree to look for lights. Nothing but fog. No stars. I moved on, trying hard to keep in a straight line. I had to spend half my time crawling under branches. I began to fall quite often. I ended up at a small pond. The same one as before? I decided to spend the night. I was wet and cold. I made a mound of leaves and twigs, and burrowed into it. I made the dogs snuggle up—the Lab along my back, the basset along my front. They were both obedient, subdued, and very warm. Someone told me later that a dog's normal temperature is several degrees higher than a human's, which makes dogs particularly good to curl up with on a cold night. In a moment of calm before I went to sleep, it suddenly occurred to me that "solo" was probably very much like this for a greater number of Outward Bound students than I'd realized. Nights of total darkness. Panic. Loss of faith in the help one *should* know is there (in their case, the pickup boat—in my case, the fact that two miles in any direction would bring me to a road). I at least had two dogs. I woke up stiff but not too cold later in the night. The stars were out. I couldn't find the Big Dipper—the only stars I knew how to use, but at least I could struggle along in a straight line following a bright one. After a half hour or so I came to a trail. Not *my* trail but sweet relief. I could stand up straight and walk. I walked happily along. Came to a pond. Different pond—bigger. End of trail. Walked the other way even more happily. Jogged a bit to get warm. The trail came into the side of a dirt road. Left or right? Guessed right. Right it was—the dirt road led to a paved road. And then to a road I knew. It turned out I'd been gone only eight hours. A mini solo. But it was the part I'd missed before.

And that, it seems to me, is the most important part of a good educational institution's effect—that you take away (perhaps unconsciously) an urge to understand the parts you missed when you were there. I don't think it's a paradox to say that the more parts you got while you were there, the more parts there are that you find you missed.

I'm sure it's clear by now that I think the Hurricane Island Outward Bound school succeeds. The staff is frank about saying that if all you want to do is learn "how to"—how to row, how to sail, how to rock-climb, et cetera—you can learn faster at specialized schools. But there is not much said about what the school intends to convey, and I can see why the staff resists trying to talk about the process. The brief descriptions I've come across are incomplete, or they are too vague or too pious, or they're written in sociological/educational jargon. I even sometimes wondered if all the staff knew what a good thing they were on to. I wondered, too, what fell into place later for the guys in my watch, and for my Dostoyevsky and Tolstoy characters—my Underground Man and my Pierre. One thing I do know is that the people I've met since who have done Outward Bound courses remember them with amazing clarity— with a clarity that amazes themselves. They—we—remember not just what we saw or what we did but how alive we felt.

Cross-Country Skiing

Before I'd ever seen a cross-country ski I used to have a recurring dream. I was on some other planet. I slipped out of a dark city, through a gap in the force field, and into a meadow. My body was changing mysteriously. It was dawn. The sky was apple-green; the air felt like a silk shirt. I had to go somewhere far away. My body was changing so that I would be able to. It grew longer and lighter. I began to run, easily but with an astonishingly powerful spring. Air came into my lungs not only through my mouth but directly through the skin of my chest. It was like slaking a deep thirst. I came to a hill. I feared that would be the end of the magic, but the new power just coiled up tighter. It made me laugh. I breasted the hill and kept on, absorbing the silver air and discharging energy downward through my calves and forward from my brow and eyes. I was acutely conscious of the trees and rocks and the air and light, and how my motion was in rhythm with them. The purpose of the journey and what lay beyond the next hill changed from dream to dream, but the original sense of my body in motion was constant and recurring.

When I finally learned how to cross-country ski, I realized these dreams had been a foretaste of sensations obtainable here and now. It wasn't like that at first, of course, nor is it like that every day now. But every so often I'm shot through with everything the dream foretold.

If you've ever had an affection for a canoe or a slender row-boat, taken pleasure in the elegance of the lines, the neat slice of the bow, the clean tuck of the stern, and felt a seed of super-stition that a boat like that is sensate and *likes* moving through the water, then you may find a particular joy in cross-country skiing: once you begin to get the motion right, the kicking and gliding and riding the driving ski with your body weight floating over it, you may find that you have swallowed your boat whole, that you are your boat moving across a lake of still air and snow.

But even the first awkward runs can have grace. The first cross-country skis I got were sturdy wide clodhoppers, not the fragile and elegant ones I have now. I was living in Iowa, where there are still strips of virgin forest by rivers and among the few hard-to-till hills and gullies. I used to bundle up and shuffle along through an oak forest, innocent of technique and wax but happy to wander alone, puffing up clouds in the motionless subzero air. The third time I went out in this forest there was a foot of snow and more falling. I jogged and poled my way along an old logging road. I reached the top of a rise and started sliding down the other side, making no more noise than a sailboat slipping through flat water.

A red fox, beautifully furred, was sitting on a stump beside the road. His tail was wrapped around his hip and across his forepaws. I could see the particular hairs of his coat. He looked at me curiously as I drifted toward him. He wasn't alarmed, I think because I wasn't making any of the moves I should have been to be advancing on him. I slid closer, and he hopped down like a cat from a sofa. About ten yards in front of me. He loped down the road—fairly casually, considering he sank in the snow up to his shoulders at each bound. I tagged along, sliding downhill after him. After a hundred yards the fox glanced around. He looked concerned that I was still with him. He upped the pace. I poled a bit and scrunched down. He glanced around again, more puzzled than alarmed. He stepped to the side of the road and let me pass by. Our eyes met. The fox pricked his ears, but there was no noise. I ghosted on down the rest of the hill, my head turned back to watch him. He came into the middle of the road and watched me, his head cocked to one side.

Skin divers tell me that they are objects of curiosity to the fish down in that silent world.

There are still patches of dream landscape to glide into quietly: a coral reef, woods muffled in a foot of snow and more falling.

•◆•

The next winter we were in Rhode Island in the cold stone cottage near Matunuck on the edge of a six- or seven-square-mile wedge of eerie second-growth woods (pine and rhododendron gone wild). The interior of the woods was dotted with glacial ponds and a few empty summerhouses. The only resemblance to Iowa was the snow, but that was wetter and coarser. But once I discovered klister waxes I was released into another winter solitude, richer for a forgotten graveyard and dilapidated stone sheep pens inaccessible to summer people because of the brambles and bull briar now snowed over. In November, before the snow, I'd got lost in these woods and spent part of a chilly night curled up in wet leaves. After it snowed, however,

I could go anywhere and be able to get home by following my tracks. I used to glide by the graveyard at dusk, the light more of a glow rising from the snow than falling from the sky. An owl sometimes followed me, winging from tree to tree, hoping to catch whatever rodent life I might scare up from underneath the snow. Once a partridge burst out of a drift at my feet, leaving a vapor trail of snow crystals hanging in front of me.

After a cold spell I was able to ski on Potter Pond, one of a series of salt ponds along the South County coast. The ice, covered with snow, was solid right up to where a narrow gut let the tide in crossways near the southern end. There the ice was suddenly cut off in a mile-long stroke as though by one slice of a knife. Going out at dusk again, I could glide right to the edge of the ice and stand quietly within twenty yards of Canada geese and black ducks paddling around in the dark seawater.

On Potter Pond part of the spell was skiing past the ghost of summer—boathouses, beached boats, and sections of dock. The neat gray-and-maroon or yellow-and-blue paint jobs, splotched with ice and blown snow, were all a shade more somber in the hard winter light.

On windy days I could take off my life jacket, hoist my parka on my ski poles, and sail downwind across the pond.

•◆•

But to do it up right, you really have to go north. I began to intrude on friends in Amherst, Massachusetts, and Putney, Vermont. It was on one of these trips that I finally saw what real cross-country skiing is. Putney was a nest of good cross-country skiers, a number of them on the U.S. team. The Putney School kids were good too, since John Caldwell was the school coach as well as the Olympic coach at that time. There are miles and miles of trails laid out for training cross-country skiers—through birchwoods and pinewoods, hayfields, and apple orchards. It was in an apple orchard that I saw a skier skimming along, each stride extending his body easily and fluidly so that for a split second at the end of each kick his upper body seemed to be flying over his forward knee. This form of skiing is more graceful than skating (which it distantly resembles), because the motions are larger and are concentrated in straight lines. I wanted that motion; I could tell that it would feel good—even better than running or skating or rowing or swimming.

Unfortunately, the winter in Rhode Island turned to rain. I tried dreaming about how to do it right (which is how I learned to downhill-ski as a kid and, later, how to shoot pheasant. I'd try for a while, then watch it done right, then hook the two together in a dream lesson).

Having had an instructive dream or two, reread John Caldwell's *The New Cross-Country Ski Book,* and jogged a bit, I entered the George Washington's Birthday Race, a southern Vermont event. Eighteen kilometers (about eleven and a half miles) from Westminster West to Putney. A crowd of four hundred or so. One hundred seeded skiers (U.S. cross-country and biathlon team members as well as college racers) lined up ahead of the mob for the mass start. At the gun the crowd yelled a collective Comanche whoop and *sprinted* forward. Like the subway at rush hour but with everyone swinging ski poles. We swept up a hill, down again, funneled across a footbridge, and then up again. And up. I fell in behind a fellow who was striding along with style. Tried to catch his rhythm. By now the crowd was strung out in double file up and around the shoulder of a hill. It looked like a procession of medieval flagellants.

On and on. I saw, or rather dimly perceived through a pulsating pinkish haze, a sign beside the trail. The sign said "Kilometer 1." I heard a far-off train whistle that turned out to be coming from my throat. But then, mysteriously, at kilometer four, it cleared up. I was skiing better than I ever had. There was a wide channel from my throat to the bottom of my lungs. The air tasted like sweet cold springwater. The birch trees were white again, the sky blue.

After the race (about an hour and a half for me) I stood for a while, bubbling with deep well-being. I felt like a potbelly stove—I was throwing off a shimmer of heat a foot in every direction. I skied back to the house where I was staying, two or three miles through the woods, still glowing with blood heat and drinking in gallons of air laced with pine trees and imminent snow.

·◆·

Although it's exciting to go to a big birthday party and have a number pinned on you and go sprinting off with a crowd and crash around the course faster than you normally would (or could), the keener and longer pleasures are solitary. There are, of course, bad days, both going out solo and going out racing. A bad day touring: packs of snowmobiles coming and going. Aside from their shrieking noise and their stink and juggernaut destruction of fences, saplings, and bird and animal life keeping warm under the snow, snowmobiles can wreck a trail for anything but another snowmobile. The engine heats up the snow. The snow refreezes into sheet ice. The next snowmobile along churns out ice chunks with its tank tread as though someone had stuck fifty cents in an ice machine. And it's not just along a narrow swath on one side of the trail. Snowmobiling for fun (I exclude practical use) is a herd sport, and snowmobile heaven is three abreast at full throttle. So you try to skate back home on the ice chunks, careen out of control, gouge your ski bottoms, hit a stone wall, and break a ski tip.

As for a bad day racing: even if you've got a piece of basic technique and some wind and muscle, there can still be a problem with snow and wax. When it's cold it's not too hard to recognize the snow type and the right basic wax. But when the snow gets wet and warm, it's a mess. Even the Finnish and Swedish run out of words for it.

One time I raced in the Putney relays. A team had lost a man, and I hopped in out of the crowd. The snow was slush. The cognoscenti were discussing what *kind* of slush it was and were blowtorching on the esoteric once-a-year waxes: hard yellow, silver klister, and mixed secret ingredients. I smeared on purple klister (all I had). The label was ambiguously translated: "For changing conditions." I got to the starting line just in time for the gun. I was dead last out of the gate, last up the hill, and last into the woods. Every time I kicked, my ski slipped backward. By the time I'd done my six-and-a-quarter-mile leg I'd raised blisters on my hands from poling. My clothes were soaked with three pounds of sweat. No quitting, because it was a relay. Near the finish there was a crowd lining the track, coming to see the hotshots. I approached this gauntlet of shame with my eyes fixed straight ahead, my cheeks burning. I slithered and lurched toward the tag line. A man pulled his wife back from crossing the track. She: "Oh, I thought they'd gone by hours ago."

How did I preen myself into this? The day before, I'd done the same distance in slightly moist snow with some speed and, I thought, some style. I'd kicked and glided along in happy solitude, almost catching up to my phantom vision of how it's done.

I tag my man. Strip off racing bib. Pull hat low over eyes. Cringing. Not one of the club, after all.

It becomes funny after a half hour. Although I can still work up a blush. And sometimes a gritty little desire to find another race, get the right wax, and whip someone's ass.

I'll dry out my peacock tail feathers some other way. Maybe a race on a dry day. Maybe. But the immediate solution is to go up to Burke Mountain and cruise around the trails. A frozen crust, not the most pleasant condition. The skis clatter over ruts, and the downhills are faster than normal. I take several nosedives at tight corners. But the wax holds somewhat up the rises. I feel better already. Halfway along the five-mile trail I come out into an open field. Across a broad valley there is a vast threatening horizon. The wind (I learn later) is blowing at almost fifty miles an hour. I can see the snow squalls coming for miles. A couple blow close by, blotting out the pine trees. A squall hits directly, and for an instant I'm breathing snow. It passes, but there's no more sun, no shadow. The sky is a milky glow, the same color as the crust. The perspective from my eyes to my ski tips is whited out. The air catches the sky and snow color. As I move along it's like floating inside a pearl. A little frightening.

Next day I sign up for a lesson. For a balm. The instructor is a young college racer. It's a bad icy day, but we have a good time. We switch the lead back and forth going around a trail so I can watch him do it right and he can see what I'm doing wrong. He allows as how my stride is pretty good (the balm), but if I'm interested in doing any racing—he pauses; I say, "Well, maybe"—then there are a few things. How to keep driving over bumps, up the rises, around turns. Also, my poles are too long, inhibiting me from getting low enough to balance forward over the driving knee. *Ah.* All good things to learn. Not just for speed but for the feel of it. We agree to meet at the next George Washington's Birthday Race.

Back home to South Newfane, Vermont, where we've migrated for this winter. I ski out late in the day on an easy flat trail that skirts a brook. The water runs black down the middle, dark green against the thick ice along the bank, and occasionally boils up in pale-green-and-white haystacks. I push hard across an open field and glide in for a rest in the shelter of the woods. The sun is going down. Two miles from home, but I feel very good. The back of my sweater, my wool hat, and my mustache are coated with the white frost of my sweat and breath. It has been a great pleasure. I wonder for a minute if some of my pleasure is sharpened because I'm afraid that these woods and fields, which should outlast me, will not. Maybe. But I felt the colors and shapes of trees in winter, the snow, and the air carrying the hard taste of the cold long before I learned to put all that in frames. And I'm sure that very early on I wondered how to travel into winter, how to enter it so that it all closed around me.

I think again of skin diving and coral reefs. I pull the ice off my mustache and knock the frost off my hat. I start home in the half-light. Going back in the tracks I've made, I feel a spurt of energy. I begin to stretch out. I pick up the tempo, balancing out over the driving ski. I feel myself catching the phantom in front of me. It feels like the old recurring dream—as if the silver air is coming through the skin of my chest and energy is uncoiling down through my legs at each stride.

POSTSCRIPT
TO CROSS-COUNTRY SKIING

Three days before what was to be my third George Washington's Birthday Race, I went over to Putney to do an eleven-kilometer trial run. The snow was fast. I had, for once, the perfect wax. It felt so good I did the trail twice. Twenty-two kilometers in an hour and twenty-two minutes—about thirteen and three-fourths miles at six minutes a mile. Jubilation.

I drove back to South Newfane. As soon as I opened the kitchen door I felt a terrible silence. I went to the next room. My wife, Jane, was holding the phone to her ear, listening. She said, "I'm coming. I'll be there tonight." Before she told me, I knew that her father had died. I hugged her while she leaned over the cradled phone. I went back to the kitchen and cried. I loved and admired Mr. Barnes. She came in and said, "Little Tracy Barnes from Manhasset."

As if mourning a son.

She packed a bag. I was to arrange a babysitter for Maud and Nell. Jane took the van. I'd find a ride to Rhode Island the next day. I can't remember who told the girls. At some point Maud, four, explained to Nell, two, that Grandpa Barnes was dead. Nell didn't know what that meant. Maud lay down on her back, closed her eyes, and held her breath.

When I got to the house in Rhode Island, Mrs. Barnes hugged me and said in my ear, "Tracy loved you so much."

I didn't think then but do now how all three generations—Jane, Maud, Mrs. Barnes—said wonderful things.

Two days later, still at the house in Rhode Island, I went for a run. It wouldn't be the last time I wanted to deal with grief by running a long way. It also wouldn't be the last time it led to a strange moment of stillness.

It was a run I'd done often, down a dirt road to a pinewoods and then through some fields. There was a broken-down stone wall between two of the fields with a large solid rock I would use as a stepping-stone to clear the wall. This time I jumped onto the rock and was held still in mid-stride. One foot was on the rock, the other out behind me. I didn't need to keep my balance. I felt weightless. It seemed that I was suspended for a long time. It could have been for a tenth of a second, it could have been longer, it could have been a vacuum in time. I was filled with light and a wordless thought from Mr. Barnes, an untranslatable comfort.

The next thing I knew I was on the dirt road, the last half mile to the house. I must have gone through the pinewoods unknowing. To tell it then wouldn't have been right. It was thirty-eight years ago. It was yesterday. It doesn't matter where it came from. I hold it unexplained and clear.

Away from New England,
Away from Saltwater and Snow

We moved to Charlottesville, Virginia. About to be thirty-four, I was surprised to find I was an assistant professor of English at the University of Virginia. After three years in Iowa and four years on an island, even a city as small as Charlottesville was culture shock. I wrote in the morning, taught in the afternoon, prepared classes late at night. I have no idea why I joined the judo club. I'd like to be able to say that because I was teaching an introductory course I thought it would be a good idea to remind myself what it was like to be a puzzled beginner. That idea came to me only later. Judo may have appeared to me as something like college wrestling, and I'd always been fascinated by John Irving's wrestling stories. Or it may have been because I saw the 1972 Summer Olympics on TV and caught one of the most astonishing and elegant human movements I've ever seen. The American heavyweight wrestler was Goliath. He outweighed the German wrestler by a hundred pounds. The American had used his weight to crush his earlier opponents. This time, after some preliminary hooking up and backing off, the American bullrushed the German. The German didn't retreat but moved into and under the American. And then suddenly the

American was over the German's head, flying through the air. The German was on the balls of his feet, his body arched back in a crescent, his arms controlling the flight of the massive American, for the moment a weightless dirigible. To learn to do that . . .

The judo club practiced in the evening two or three times a week for about two and a half hours. The beginners first learned how to fall. We'd throw ourselves in the air and try to land more or less painlessly, distributing the impact and using our arms to whack the mat as a counterforce exactly when we hit. Then we practiced throws. The sensei, a powerful and perfectly proportioned African American, was a former Marine 205-pound judo champion. He spent most of his time with the black belts while the assistant instructors taught us the basics. When we began sparring (*randori*), he got interested.

Judo translates from Japanese as "gentle way." Yes and no. Sparring with a black belt was like a dance, and getting thrown was the final and sometimes most graceful step. Sparring with ex–football players was more rough-and-tumble.

After a while I began to get the idea. The idea is that the two judo players are contained in a hemisphere made up of arc after arc. You have to sense which arc your opponent is moving along and accelerate him through it. To do this there are leg sweeps, trips, hip throws, and once in a great while something like the German's arc, but done on your back and using your legs and feet to send your opponent flying. A clean throw at the end of which your opponent lands flat on his back is ruled *ippon*—translation: whole bottle. Match over. Most often a thrown judo player twists and avoids *ippon,* and the match goes on as grappling on the mat. Three ways to win: control your opponent on his back for thirty seconds, get a joint hold that will dislocate the joint or break a bone (either the ref stops the match before this happens or the player taps out), or get a choke hold on the carotid artery. The choked player will either tap out or pass out.

By the time the spring term started I was of two minds. I was hooked on the chess-match aspect: for every throw there is a counter-throw, and for every counter-throw . . . perhaps not ad infinitum but a dizzying progression. I also achieved an occasional *ippon*. I kept two ACE bandages in my locker, and they moved from joint to joint. I didn't mind that—part of the dues. What I *did* mind was that I began thinking about judo obsessively. Bicycling to work, walking the dogs, taking a shower, or—most intrusively—while sitting at my desk, trying to write a novel.

I'm glad I didn't quit then. There were two moments I'm pleased to think about. One was when our sensei came to class fired up. He lined us up and said that if we wanted to get better we had to want it harder. "Messing around with each other ain't gonna do it. You got to want to go through me. I'm the man. Anybody? Come on now."

Sometimes my common sense floats away. I said, "Yes."

I had been practicing one particular throw over and over. It took us both by surprise. But on his way down he was not only twisting but starting his first grappling move. He got me on my back and pressed his chest against mine with all his weight, making it hard to breathe. I tried one thing, then another. I stopped to think. He whispered in my ear, "Come on, white boy. Don't give up." Another two attempts at escape and the thirty seconds were up.

Perhaps because of that one throw, he picked me to go with the team he sent to a tournament. My third match of the day was against another 176-pounder, though he looked smaller than me. He turned in to me as if to try *osotogari* (major hip throw). I thought I would get him in a bear hug and throw him sideways. My arms closed around . . . nothing. He was gone. The next thing I knew, we were on the mat. He was behind me, working the edge of his hand into my neck. I tucked my chin in, but the next thing I knew the ref was saying, "Can you tell me your name, son?" It came to me slowly. "Okay, son. Just lie there and take a few breaths."

I didn't want to end on that note, so I went to two more club sessions, got in a decent foot sweep, and hung up my *gi*.

I was working at writing, teaching, and preparing classes. Ten hours Monday through Friday, a few hours of writing Saturday. I still needed something physical. I saw an announcement: the JFK Memorial Fifty-Mile Hike/Run. President Kennedy had once said that every U.S. Marine should be able to march fifty miles in one day. Anyone game?

Fifty Miles

I mentioned the JFK hike/run to John Rowlett, whom I first met as a sparring partner, a black belt who'd been the 176-pound champion of Texas. It turned out he had more strings to his bow. He was getting a Ph.D. in English literature, and at the same time was the editor of *Birds of Texas,* one of the bibles of ornithologists, since the state has a huge variety of both North American and Central American birds.

John said yes. He was in good shape from judo, and the summer before, he'd followed a bird in Mexico all day, for what he was pretty sure was fifty miles.

I put in five weeks of daily jogging or walking for an hour or so, mostly after dark. My route included a golf course bordered by wide stands of trees. I didn't see wildlife but heard it. I was reminded of a Faulkner sentence: "He went on down the hill, toward the dark woods within which the liquid silver voices of the birds called unceasingly—the rapid and urgent beating of the urgent and quiring heart of the late spring night."

As is often the case, the training at long, slow distances— the mind drift brought on by an easy lope—was the pleasure. The actual event rated a notch lower—a satisfaction reached with more jaggedness.

The fifty-mile course started with a fifteen-mile section of the Appalachian Trail in Maryland. A gang of runners ran up the first hill. We trotted, passing those who slowed down to hike. After about ten miles John Rowlett stepped off the trail to piss. He reported that he'd pissed blood. He added, "My old sensei told us it was better not to wear a jockstrap. Maybe I should have."

"How do you feel?"

"I'll go on for a bit."

"My wife is meeting us at mile fifteen. I've got a spare pair of jockey shorts in our van."

But at mile fifteen Rowlett decided to slow down. We were now starting an eighteen-mile section of the C&O Canal towpath. My wife said she'd meet us at one of the canal locks nine miles farther along.

Rowlett changed into the jockey shorts but didn't want to risk jogging. As it turned out, it wasn't a serious problem, but it was alarming.

It began to rain. One of the advantages of keeping a messy family car is that there's always something that comes in handy. In this case, an umbrella and a poncho. Rowlett opted for the poncho. The runners in shorts and T-shirts got soaked and chilled. Those who put on rain jackets sweated so much that they also got soaked and chilled. I recommend an umbrella. I was sweating, but the breeze dried me. When one arm got tired, I switched. I decided to jog for a couple of miles, then alternate brisk walking with jogging. After a while I was alone except for a walker far in front of me and a jogger behind me. I could see each of them at a distance. The towpath afforded a long view. What was odd was that the jogger didn't seem to catch up, and I didn't seem to be gaining on the walker. This was distracting. I distracted myself further by looking at my watch too often. I was reckoning to jog for ten minutes, walk for fifteen minutes. I'd look at my watch after what seemed a long while. Only five minutes had gone by. I also lost track of the overall time. No idea how far to mile twenty-four. I was suspended in a zone of no time. I decided to pass the walker in front of me, to hell with looking at my watch. That done, I walked fast enough to lose the walker. The jogger behind me disappeared. I jogged and walked with no one in sight. I finally saw our red van. I jogged and jogged, but it seemed not to get closer. Walked. My wife came back to walk alongside in an encouraging way. I sat down by the van and ate a handful of peanuts and wheat germ, and drank cranberry juice. I thought, *Not even halfway.* That was the low point. Rowlett was there. He'd backtracked to mile fifteen and thumbed a ride. He urged me to get going. He said, "One of us should do it." *Right.*

After a mile or so I felt good again. The food kicked in, and I also got a rhythm. When I walked I sang to myself, show tunes, Gregorian chant, even "Hush, little baby, don't you cry." When I got through all the verses I could remember, I jogged again. Jogged until it felt like it was time to walk.

Before I knew it I was at a canal lock and a lockkeeper's house. I crossed the footbridge over the canal and sat down on a stump.

A couple of boys came out of the house and handed me a mug of coffee. That cup of instant coffee with sweetened condensed milk is one of my clearest memories of something tasting so good that I closed my eyes with pleasure. The combination of an ounce or so of condensed milk, the caffeine, and the kindness made me feel like Popeye after a can of spinach. Off at a trot.

The rain stopped. I missed the pattering on my umbrella. At a farther lock there was a sign directing contestants to a two-lane blacktop. A race official handed me a plastic tube. When it got dark, I was to give it a squeeze, and it would glow bright green to alert cars going by.

Jane had cleverly found this spot. I changed my shirt and got rid of the umbrella. Only seven more miles. After a fifteen-minute jog I asked some men on a porch how far to Antietam. "Oh, seven or eight miles." I knew they were wrong, but I got discouraged anyway. Farther along there was a line of packed cars, a way station of friends and relatives of hikers/runners.

"How far?"

"Three-point-eight miles. The last half-mile's the driveway to a school. The finish line is at the school."

This was too much encouragement. I trotted, but then I had to slow down. At last the turn onto the driveway. People were waving flashlights. It was now dark enough so that the light made me night-blind for a bit. But then I could see—I'd been here before—this was the Saint James School. I scored a goal here years ago in a soccer game; the next spring I won a bronze in the javelin. I thought I could sprint. I managed a barely noticeable acceleration.

The finish line wasn't at the top of the driveway—what seemed to me the sensible and obvious place—but fifty yards farther into a parking lot. I felt put-upon. And then: *That's it?*

It wasn't until I was back at the motel and soaking in a hot bath that I began to get rid of the mood of anticlimax.

On the ride back the next day, John Rowlett looked out the windows and said, "The dogwood are adumbrating the wild cherry."

I wasn't sure exactly what *adumbrating* meant, but that sentence struck me as a note to end on.

The next day I went to the UVA track just to loosen up. I ran into a student of mine who was on the track team. He asked me if I'd done the fifty miles. He shook my hand. A teammate of his came over, a distance runner. My student said, "This professor just did the JFK fifty-miler."

The distance runner said, "What was your time?"

I shaved off the twenty-five minutes I'd taken for lunch at mile twenty-four. I said, "Ten hours."

The distance runner barked a laugh and said, "Room for improvement."

My student was embarrassed. I thought it was funny. A reflexive blurt.

I later learned from a newspaper account that only about half of the entrants finished. The last finisher came in after seventeen hours. The man who won, a UVA law student, ran the whole way at seven minutes per mile. That is amazing. I was in the middle of the pack, somewhere between the dogwood adumbrating the wild cherry and room for improvement.

Farewell to Fox Island

My wife, our two daughters, and I went back to Fox Island in June. It became clear that it wasn't going to work as a place to spend the summer. By the time we got through the first list of chores it was well into July and almost time to start battening down the island for the winter. We were both writing novels, but any money from those was still in the future. Now even the tiny mortgage payments on the island seemed an extravagance. I also realized that my favorite season on the bay had been fall.

We spent that summer readying the house to show to a real-estate agent, and inviting those friends who'd liked being on the island and were good at it.

The most adept and welcome was David Plimpton. He'd drive from New York late on Friday night, unload his kayak and paddle to the island, and crank up the work skiff and go back to his car to get two bags of groceries, a case of beer, and his Labrador, an old friend of my own Lab. Plimpton was good at fixing things, seeing how to rerig the davits at the end of the dock, how to shore up the seawall. Even Lenny Chesney said he was salty.

Best of all, he liked poking into anything that looked interesting. One day he and I took the work skiff into Wickford

Harbor. A large double-decker barge was tied up at the town dock, listing badly toward mid-channel. A man was pacing back and forth on top, having an argument with the harbormaster. The man was actually having several arguments. The second argument was with the man who owned the cinderblock building around which the barge owner had run a cable to keep his barge from sliding into the channel. The cable was eating into the corner of the building. The other arguments were harder to follow. The only snatch of them I caught was about a pump.

David and I asked if we could come aboard. The barge owner was glad to be distracted. Aside from the lively arguments, what attracted David and me was a steel lifeboat that had apparently come from a larger vessel. "S.S. *Greensburg*" was stenciled near her bow.

The barge owner told the three men on the dock that he had to confer with David and me. This puzzled the men enough to give the barge owner a time-out.

The barge owner's story was that he'd had a deal to open a floating restaurant on her. The barge owner had arranged to have her towed to Newport. She'd sprung a leak during the tow. The man with the towboat brought her to Wickford, hoping to get her to a boatyard, but she had taken on too much water to get there, so the owner had tied her up at the town dock while he went to look for an auxiliary bilge pump. He didn't have any cash, and no one would take his check. He was back on board now to defend her.

The owner of the cinder-block building was threatening to hacksaw the cable. The harbormaster didn't want the barge to sink and slide into the channel, which would block traffic from two marinas. His idea was to tow her out into the bay before she took on even more water, run her aground anywhere but in his harbor. A third man was trying either to collect a debt or to get some cash up front for renting an auxiliary bilge pump.

There was more to it, but that was pretty much the state of play.

I fell in love with the lifeboat. Not a lovely boat—a kind of thick-waisted peapod—but something about her appealed to me. I asked if the lifeboat might be for sale.

"What'll you offer?"

"What'll you take?"

I can't remember the exact figures, but we went back and forth until we hit on a price—maybe two hundred dollars. I said I'd go back to the island, get my checkbook, cash it in town, and come back. The barge owner was afraid the man on the dock would hacksaw the cable if we left.

Plimpton had his wallet with him. Between us, we had a third in cash, and the barge owner took Plimpton's check for the rest.

It took all three of us just to slide the lifeboat off the roof, even though the barge was tilting severely toward the channel.

The barge owner took up his negotiations with the man on the dock, apparently successfully, since I later learned the barge owner got a bilge pump and got the barge to float enough to move her to a boatyard.

Plimpton and I got back to the island with whatever supplies we'd come for—plus the lifeboat. One of the details I'd liked about her was the additional single oarlock just to the right of the pointed stern. It was for a *steering* oar. The other detail I liked was that she was painted royal purple.

At that time we owned the reluctant inboard, a new work skiff, the old rowing skiff, and a canoe I hadn't been able to resist at a garage sale. The evening before, my wife overheard

Plimpton touting the pleasures of kayaking and offering to find me one secondhand. My wife had suggested that it was time to reduce the boat inventory.

As we approached the island with the lifeboat in tow, it occurred to me that neither the extra stern oarlock nor the royal-purple paint job would do for her what they did for me. I tried to think of an opening gambit.

"I didn't buy a kayak." Try again.

"The girls will love her." Warmer.

"We need a really safe boat for the girls, and she's a *life*boat."

A family friend is often the answer. Jane was waiting on the dock. She lit into Plimpton. "Why didn't you stop him? You know what he's like. He's like Toad in *The Wind in the Willows*."

I said, "I think you mean Water Rat," but luckily she didn't hear me. Plimpton, six-foot-three and a former 195-pound college wrestler, looked enormously sheepish. Jane was mollified.

The lifeboat was so heavy we couldn't haul her onto the beach, so we anchored her. After Plimpton cooked supper and I washed the dishes, I took her for a twilight row. She was so heavy it took ten hard strokes to get her moving, but once under way she kept going. Her *theoretical* hull speed, given her sixteen-foot length, was five or six knots, but she didn't seem to like more than three and a half knots, just a hair more than four miles per hour. She was happy to do that without asking for more than long, steady strokes on eight-foot oars. I rowed her up and down the bay, sometimes with Plimpton, sometimes solo, sometimes trolling for fish, sometimes just for fun.

A four-acre island with only a one-lung diesel generator for electricity, with no heat except for driftwood fires, and no phone turned out to be a hard sell. It wasn't until two years later that the right sort of eccentrics turned up—an ex-RAF officer who'd built his own gyroplane. He was married to an ex-nun. They had the necessary big dog, a German shepherd named Satan.

We sold the island, threw in the work skiff, sold the reluctant inboard. I kept the canoe and small skiff. Plimpton bought the lifeboat, by then repainted bright orange. He wanted to take her to his parents' house in Osterville on Cape Cod. Could we find a boat trailer with a winch? She weighed so much that four strong men could barely lift her. Plimpton said, "We can row her."

I set to planning the route with a chart and tide tables. I like the beer-bottle method. If you put an empty well stoppered beer bottle in at point A, will the tides and prevailing winds take the bottle to point B? If we put the *Greensburg* in at dawn, at the top of the tide, nine miles from the mouth of Narragansett Bay, the first half of the dumping tide would help move her beyond Narragansett Pier. Then the second half of the ebb coming out of Long Island Sound and across Rhode Island Sound would help get her to Cuttyhunk, the southernmost of the Elizabeth Islands. At that time—in theory, about noon—the tide would change and help the *Greensburg* up the chain of islands (Cuttyhunk, Nashawena, Naushon). The tidal current between the Elizabeth Islands to the west and Martha's Vineyard to the east is swift. The bonus would be that the southwest wind usually starts to blow at about noon. Also in theory, the *Greensburg* would breeze past Woods Hole at about teatime. The short trip from Woods Hole to Osterville wouldn't be a problem.

Plimpton and I thought of two more bonuses. He thought that since the Cuttyhunk–to–Woods Hole leg would be downwind, why not rig a sail? We put in a thick plank from gunwale to gunwale and jigsawed a hole for a stubby mast, made a square-rigged sail from a tarp. That would mean that the rowers would have to row only six hours or so to Cuttyhunk, then get a rest for the next three or four hours before rowing along the south edge of Cape Cod to Osterville, another several hours. If that last leg was hard, pull up on a beach and picnic on cranberry juice and Triscuits.

My idea was to recruit a third rower. Jack Lawrence, who was running a red crab–processing plant near Galilee, Rhode Island, was an ex–college rower and had done survival training in Panama when he was in the military. He said yes.

With three men, we could rotate the rowing, two hours on, one hour off.

Checklist: chart, 5 eight-foot oars (you never know), juice and Triscuits, life preservers, anchor and chain, and fifty feet of line . . .

On the eve of setting out, I felt odd. By ten at night I had a 103-degree fever. My wife told me later I was delirious, that I kept sitting up in bed and saying, "Where are my men? Let them in. They're trying to get in." And later, "Where's the beer bottle?"

When I woke up, it was noon. They'd left without me. Mutiny! But Jack had to be at the crab plant the next day, and there wouldn't be a conjunction of a dawn high tide and a Sunday or Saturday for a long time. At dawn they'd told Jane they could wait another hour. She told them to go before I woke up. She was right. I would have acted unreasonably.

I wasn't mad at them. I was glad when they phoned my mother-in-law to say they made Woods Hole just before the tide turned against them. But I felt a shame I couldn't dislodge. I'd rowed the *Greensburg* for miles and miles, and now she was gone. I tried to redeem my weakness by paddling my canoe on the bay, sometimes all the way to Narragansett, sometimes in stormy weather. I entered a six-mile canoe race down the Pettaquamscutt River with a Polish Zen Buddhist as bowman. One hour, middle of the pack. It was exercise, not an adventure. I would need something else for redemption.

Winter Outward Bound

The next time you're out skiing or snowshoeing or just taking a walk in the snow, look at the nearest snowdrift and consider how you would do if you had to spend the night in it. You might ask yourself, *Would I freeze to death?* Okay, we'll add a sleeping bag rated to zero degrees Fahrenheit. *How miserable will I be?* I certainly asked myself that. I didn't think of asking, *Will it be, in its peculiar way, fun?*

Last winter I spent eleven days outdoors in Maine, taking an Outward Bound survival course. Two days and nights I was alone in my own snow cave. I was sure I wouldn't freeze to death—I had wool clothes and a good sleeping bag. I wasn't miserable at all, although I was nervous about being miserable. It was fun—partly. It was certainly satisfying and instructive.

The course I went through was administered by the Hurricane Island Outward Bound. Its summer operation is on the Maine coast, but this one took place in the Mahoosuc Range in western Maine. It was shorter than the standard twenty-six-day course, but had the three standard elements: training expedition, solo, and final expedition.

•◆•

TRAINING

On the eve of the first day we gathered in the Sunday River Inn. We'd been told to bring wool clothes and a flashlight, knife, and sunglasses. Outward Bound provided everything else for the next eleven days: Sorel boots with felt liners, snow-shoes, touring skis, sleeping bags, a tent (only for the first night), chamois face masks, pots and pans, one wood saw, one snow saw, a pile of food, and frame packs with which to lug it all.

The first day we set out from the bottom of the ski slope. Downhill skiers flit past us in a rainbow of bright ski jackets and stretch pants. They gawk at us, a gang of sad sacks in baggy woollies, and we are eager to disappear into the woods. The packs, ranging from forty to sixty pounds, about a third of the weight of the backpacker, are awkward. We crab up the slope on snowshoes, the touring skis lashed vertically.

Our senior instructor, Chris, mumbles that we shouldn't mind. He adds, "This bit is always somewhat embarrassing." We lurch on in a clatter of pots, pans, and skis. We try not to stop for breath until we're out of sight.

Chris and the two young women lead the way, then the four men, ranging from a twentysomething up to age thirty-eight (I'm the oldest). Alex, the assistant instructor, brings up the rear. He has the busiest time. Several people fall, some more than once, and they need a helping hand to get up out of the deep snow. Once in the woods one of the men catches the top of his skis on an overhead branch and does a back dive into the snow. He's buried. His snowshoes are stuck edgewise, and he's anchored by his backpack and lashed skis. Alex fits ski poles into his hands and helps him plant them. Once he's up, Alex recommends that he brush off all the snow before it melts from his body heat. "Wet is what you don't want to be."

It was probably a three-hour hike, but it seemed longer. For several people this first day was the worst part. I suspect it's part of Outward Bound pedagogy to start each session with a jolt. Certainly the awkwardness of the first time on snowshoes is tiring. And there's anxiety—What have I got myself into? Lisa, one of two high-school girls, later told me that as soon as she strapped her pack on she was horrified. She felt both burdened and unbalanced. She was sure that if she fell behind she would give up. So she hustled to the front and stayed there, trying not to think about how long this was going to go on. It wasn't until day two or three that most of us came to admire whoever invented snowshoes. (Some form of snowshoes and skis have been unearthed in Russia dating from the Neolithic era. It was the same Stone Age people who invented boats and knots. Claude Lévi-Strauss loves these pre-literate inventors.)

The first night we slept in a huge tent. There was a stiff breeze. I was happy to be sheltered. At some point I woke up. I realized I had to piss, which involves unzipping my two-layer sleeping bag, thawing my boots against my chest until I can fit them on. I manage not to wake anyone up. I find my snowshoes. It's snowing, and there's a dark glow to the night. I wonder, not for the first or last time, about where the light comes from. But uppermost in my mind is a resolution not to drink four cups of soup at supper.

The first two days everyone is busy with this kind of minor-but-crucial adjustment. Another one is the choice between sleeping with your boots between the inner and outer layer of your sleeping bag, in which case you have to hold them against your body to thaw them, or keeping them in the inner bag, where you are more apt to roll onto them and wake yourself up. Then there's dealing with boot laces, gaiters, snowshoe bindings, pack straps . . . And once on the trail, the constant striptease to keep from pouring sweat. Keeping dry is vital. But soon enough all this fussing becomes easier and then automatic.

Chris and Alex take turns at conveying basic instructions, usually around the evening campfire. (1) *Eat.* We each eat five thousand to six thousand calories a day. Seeds and nuts and root vegetables, but also peanut-butter cups, meat, and cocoa. I still lost five pounds in eleven days. Part of it was exertion, but another part was that our bodies turned up their thermostats. By the end of the trip you could stand next to someone and feel the heat radiating. (2) *Drink.* You need at least ten cups of liquid to digest all this food. Dehydrated bodies lose heat alarmingly fast. (3) *Don't get cold. Well, uh, sure.* But it turns out that cold is subtler than your senses are used to, and once you get really cold, you tend to do less about it. So keep checking.

Once we loved our snowshoes, Chris switched us to skis. Those people used to downhill skiing had to adjust to skating and doing step turns rather than trying to christie. Lisa and I had both done cross-country skiing, but after my time at Hurricane Island in a boat with ten rowers, I kept my trap shut—well, mostly shut. I let Lisa offer the helpful hints.

After a few hours we stopped for lunch. Chris got out a couple of topographical maps and compasses. He gave a brief chat on where we were on the map and what we could see around us and what it looked like on the map.

"Right," he said suddenly. "I'll meet you there." He pointed to a spot on the map, surrounded by closely serried contour lines. I know enough to know that meant steep and, in this case, up.

"At that notch there?"

"Yes. You call it a notch, do you? Saddle, col, notch. In Scotland they call it a *bilach*." One of the nice quirks of Outward Bound instruction is to undercut the notion that naming things gives you any power. You can pronounce *glissade* or *cwm* and still be useless at getting anywhere.

We watch Chris winkle off through the trees, not in the right direction. We finish lunch and put on our skis. Alex waves good-bye and says he'll see us tomorrow.

I take the map-reading too seriously, want to study it at length. Several other people take it too lightly. Fortunately, Walden emerges as navigator. He has a good eye for the shape of the land and how it relates to the flat map in his hand. We set out for Jordan Notch.

At first the mohair strips on our ski bottoms keep us from sliding backward, but soon we have to go back and forth in long traverses, then herringbone. Finally, the way up is so steep we have to sidestep. An ABC of uphill skiing.

At last we find Chris, who's built a fire and offers us a pot of cocoa. Then he suggests we move on to find a campsite lower down.

After the ABC of up, there's *D* for down. It's one thing to ski down a well-packed open slope, your feet in stiff boots clamped to the skis, and using steel edges to cut your turns. It's another thing to go down through a forest in deep snow, in your soft boots with only a toehold on the skinny skis. There's also the pack frame jutting a half-foot over your head. Just when you thought you'd neatly ducked under a branch, you hear a *thwonk* behind your head. You end up on your ass. The snow is deep, so it's not painful. It's like being thrown in judo by a kindly black belt.

After the steep part there's pleasure. On the gentler downhill slope there's time to plan a zigzag course. It's like dancing through the birch trees in a slow waltz.

We have a long move the next day, but everyone's cheerful. We also don't need management. Without orders, someone gathers wood, someone starts the fire and boils water, someone finds the oatmeal canister.

My pack is heavier since we redistributed the loads, but it rides better. When we get out of the woods and onto a logging trail I find I can kick and glide even with a full pack. It's not full cross-country style, in which every stride feels like a wingbeat, but there's some grace. We reach more open ground with a view to the north of the higher hills we're going to tour. The sky is deep blue; there's only a little loose snow on top of the crust. Breathing is like drinking from a spring.

Lisa, who had to grit her teeth the first day, is now enjoying herself. Even Lon, our Texan, who'd had trouble on skis at first—his pack seemed to have an impish will of its own, pushing him forward, then tilting him back—is keeping his balance, keeping the pace.

By mid-afternoon there is general sagging but then rejoicing when we reach the long glide into the valley that is to be our next campsite. Lon, Lisa, and David are sent off to build a three-person igloo, a step up from a snow cave.

The next day we climb to Jake's Notch, higher and steeper but surprisingly easier. On the long level stretch into camp I make the mistake of going flat out on my skis. I end up pouring sweat. Marcy, the other high-school girl, Walden, and I are sent off to try our hand at an igloo. I'm giddy from a couple of miles of deep breathing the clean, cold air. I propose a grand igloo plan. We cut snow blocks with the tails of our skis, build it up in spirals. When we get to the last small circle at the top, the whole thing caves in. We stare at it. We look to the west, where the sun is sinking into the White Mountains.

Marcy and I both say, "Shit."

Walden pokes at the rubble. He says, "Oh, well. Nome wasn't built in a day."

Not bad for a darkening afternoon in the Maine woods. My beard has icicles in it. They sound like wind chimes when I laugh. Marcy points out that we can sleep in the hole in the snow we've made. Walden and I say that it looks like a grave. But she's right. We put deadwood across the top and use the igloo blocks as roof tiles. By the time we're done the moon is up. I climb into the pit to do some housekeeping, and also because I've suddenly got even colder. Marcy and Walden go for a quick ski by midnight.

When they get back I apologize for my overambitious igloo plan, for being grumpy about being wet and cold. No problem. And so to bed. They put me in the middle to make sure I'll be warm.

• ◆ •

TWO-DAY SOLO

I'd had a wonderful time by myself for four September days on a tiny island off the coast of Maine, daydreaming; gathering rose hips, sea-urchin roe, and mussels; sleeping on a bed of leaves and pine needles; and watching herons. This is to be a shorter solo, but the question of shelter is more pressing. Chris mentions that there's a snowstorm coming, probably by evening. I'm only a mile or so from camp, but the feeling is—and is meant to be—one of isolation.

I stand still for a while, looking around. There's no wind, no movement, just a gray day. After a moment I notice there's a touch of rose in the young birch trees. I startle myself when I clear my throat.

I ski around, looking for a place to rest. I get lucky—there's a large fallen tree; the thick base of the trunk is propped up by the roots. I clear the snow away, using a snowshoe as a shovel. I find enough long sticks to make a lean-to, tile the roof with blocks of snow. I serve them onto the roof with the tail of a ski. It takes more time and energy than I'd thought. It's mid-afternoon. I eat a carrot and saltines, save the raisins. I climb inside to check the roof—still some gaps. My leather mittens are oozing yellow water again, but this is a help—when I slap more snow on top, it'll be wet, and then it'll freeze, making a more stable roof.

I move my pack inside. My stove is a #10 can with holes in the side, my pot a #10 can without holes. I gather twigs and light a fire. Fill the pot with snow. I lay the snowshoes down as bedsprings, some spare clothes as the mattress. I turn around when I hear a *plop*. My stove is too near the mouth of my shelter, and the roof is melting. I manage to get my mittens on and move both cans. Didn't the guy in the Jack London story make the same mistake? Built his fire under a tree, and the snow on the branches fell and put it out. I should have known better.

It's dark. I make soup by throwing in a bouillon cube, a

carrot, half an onion, and half a potato. I have to keep feeding twigs in through the holes. It takes forever until the vegetables are soft. Worth the wait. I open the one tin—it's olive drab, Army surplus, stenciled "Chocolate Nut Roll." With an effort of will, I eat only half.

It begins to snow. This is a good thing. It'll insulate the roof even more. I'm feeling snug, even smug, as I crawl into my sleeping bag.

Just as I'm falling asleep I feel a warm breath on my cheek. I lie very still. This fallen tree makes such a good den, something else might be holed up here. A bear? The space is too small, but a porcupine . . . I arm myself with a ski pole. My flashlight is dim from the cold—I should have kept it in my sleeping bag, along with my boots. Nothing under the tree trunk, but I feel warm air. At last I realize that it's warmth from the decomposing bits of leaves and twigs under the armpit, so to speak, of the uprooted tree. I curl up peacefully.

The next day passes in a lovely waking dreaminess. It has snowed six inches of several varieties of flakes. The weather was changing through the night and keeps changing all day. From placid white to a gusty blue-and-gray afternoon to a quiet gray twilight. I haven't done much during the day except stroll around. I did whittle a wooden spoon, but otherwise just looked. I considered trees. I watched the moon rise. Behind a moving curtain of clouds I found the Big Dipper, the only constellation I know except for Orion.

I wake up at first light. I hear a noise. A crackling or even crunching. Someone, something, walking in the snow? I hold still, not breathing. The noise stops. Maybe nothing. When I breathe again I hear it. After a few cycles of holding my breath and then breathing again, it becomes clear that the noise is my own breath soughing across the edge of my sleeping-bag hood.

Okay, two embarrassing false alarms. I laugh at myself once, stretch, and then curl up peacefully.

When I wake up again the day is undecided between high blue sky and low gray clouds. I decide to sleep until this question of color is resolved, but Alex arrives on skis to roust me. "Just follow my tracks." When I get to the logging trail, I catch up to the rest of the clan.

We are happy to see one another. It seems a long time. We would have hugged, but we were on skis.

When we glided into camp, Chris had a fire going. He'd been all the way back to the lodge and brought an orange for each of us. We'd had almost the same experience, hour for hour. Lisa and I had heard the same owls. When the sun was out we'd all worshipped it. Marcy actually washed her hair. Lon washed a shirt. We'd all tensed up at noises that turned out to be nothing. We'd been sown like seeds the length of the valley, all sprouting similar thoughts. For the rest of the trip there was a marked increase in energetic tenderness for one another.

·◆·

FINAL EXPEDITION

There is something of a bluff to the Outward Bound formulation of "final expedition." Chris gave us the official version: "It's up to you now; I'm just one of the party." But really his heart was set on Old Speck. It's not a major peak, only 4,200 feet, including a fire tower. Chris told us that the group before us had to turn back. We all agreed. We found it appealing that Chris, an experienced explorer, was so eager. I found out later that he'd written a book, *A Rockclimber's Guide to the Crags of Kenya*.

It takes us two days to move up to the notch from which we'll climb. The afternoon before Old Speck, Chris and Alex ask Walden, Lisa, and me to go with them to look at the steep side to see if it's too hard. Old Speck has a long slope on the north side, a steep side on the south, a drumlin.

We have to kick one tip of a snowshoe into the wall of snow, then kick in the other a step higher. Then do it again. We get pretty high up, but after a couple of hours it's clear that the short, steep route would actually take longer.

When we turn back we see that we're on top of a series of ledges, each with about a fifteen-foot vertical wall, then a short shelf, then another wall. There are some evergreens—spruce, I think, but it's hard to tell, since the branches are covered with snow. Alex says "Geronimo" and jumps. His fall is softened first by the tips of the snowy branches, then by the deep snow on the ledge. We follow him. We land and tumble into the snow, shake ourselves, and jump off the next ledge. On the third jump Walden breaks the edge of his snowshoe. Alex examines it, takes out his knife, and makes a long scarf joint. He cuts off a good length of his bootlace and binds the two pieces with a six-inch-long fisherman's knot. When I say something about this resourceful bit of repair, Alex shrugs. He says, "My full-time job is carpentry."

He'd told us earlier that he'd been Special Forces in Vietnam. After he was discharged he became a Quaker. The British Outward Bound instructors tend to be from northern England or Scotland. The American instructors are often repentant military.

After the broken snowshoe, we go down more carefully. Not nearly as much fun.

The day of the climb we get up at four, because we'll have to turn back at two in the afternoon. We're on snowshoes, with light packs—an extra sweater, long johns, and a sleeping bag just in case. We hike along the base for an hour or so, then start up, at first a gentle slope and then steep. Even on the easier side, there's an almost vertical part that requires kicking in the front of the snowshoe and going step by slow step. It's like rock climbing in terms of working hard for each foot up, but without the terror.

Over the lip of the steep part there is a more gentle slope. We're no longer scrambling, just shuffling along through head-high trees that glitter with hoarfrost. Some of the trees are laced together by frost arches, and on these arches there is an even more delicate sort of hoarfrost that falls in glitter as we brush past.

Another slope up. The trees thin even more, and the frost and snow are so bright we put on sunglasses. Now we feel the north wind. We tuck our chins in, until, one by one, we see the fire tower. Our crowing is carried off by the wind.

We stay long enough to drink a thermos full of hot grape juice and for a few people to take a look from the tower. My fingers are so cold I can't get my snowshoes off. My mittens, wet from scrabbling up, stiffen in the wind. But the satisfaction squares any effort or chill. The brilliance of the frost garden is an unaccountable bonus—a brilliant, eerie delight as we start back through it, and I take my sunglasses off to let the frost trees flare up against the scorched blue sky. It is almost too beautiful to bear.

Even before we're off the edge of the top, we unwind into

careless trail chat, the loose-muscle relief of going down in snowshoes.

After swinging down the steep part, grabbing branches like orangutans with webbed feet, we lope and straggle all along our trail. It's pleasant to be a little apart in the dark green woods—tired out but warmed up again—a little dazed, the inner eye still dazzled. I find myself humming "We Are Climbing Jacob's Ladder."

There have been moments when we had to gather our strength or our wits, but no one had to be coaxed out of despair, and this general goodwill probably played a part. (When I was in a twelve-man whaleboat for a twenty-six-day course eight years ago, there was much more surliness during the first part of the expedition. There were a few men aboard who thought I was a sonofabitch, and I thought they were assholes, two of them useless assholes.) Perhaps age has mellowed me; I think everyone on this trip is just fine, and something like this sympathy is true for all of us.

The other reason, I figure, is that we caught on fairly quickly that our own pleasure and well-being were framed by a fairly harsh environment; that if you're a group of eight you can keep warm, but if you're alone you can get very cold; that if you have to build a shelter, it takes four times longer alone than it does with one other person; and that if you're skiing or snowshoeing by yourself, you're always breaking trail, and in a group of eight, there'll be seven times you don't have to. And these are only the most obvious simplicities.

The next day we climb Sunday River Whitecap in the morning: a piece of cake. It is a grand panorama—the White Mountains to the southwest, Mount Washington visible in vast detail—Maine flattening out invitingly to the other side past a few solitary cones, Tumbledown and Sugarloaf. And we are so stoked with combustible energy that we have a cheerful snowball fight back at camp. Then we pack up and hike to our last campsite, near Screw Auger Falls, where we will be picked up the next morning.

Around the last campfire we hold a pleasant debriefing. It can be a little bristly, but we are mostly all goodwill and praise.

The conversation does bring out some funny first impressions. There is admiration for Lisa and Marcy, who've become Valkyries. Lisa thinks the older people turned out okay. She says to me, "When I first saw you back at the inn before we started—you know, you sitting there smoking your pipe and reading Thomas Hardy—I couldn't imagine you coming along and being any fun. Then I thought, *Well, give him a chance—he's no older than Robert Redford.*"

I ask Chris how he would like to spend his time, if he could do whatever he wanted. More serious expeditions? He says he intends to explore some lava caves he's come across in Rwanda, but he is happy doing Outward Bound courses. He says, "Not all the courses are as pleasant as this one, but I usually finish them feeling good. Feeling quite fit, among other things. I haven't been strained this trip—nor have you, I imagine—but on serious expeditions you sometimes have to struggle to get through, and you end up pretty worn down. Once every year or so is fine. But I'm quite happy spending most of the year like this."

We talked about high points and low points, and a few odd points, an example of an odd point being the day the toilet paper got wet and we had to use snowballs. (Not as bad as you'd expect.)

Lon asks if the way he's known us for eleven days is the way we are. Marcy answers, "Sure, the Marcy you see is the Marcy you get." Lon gives the most interesting answer when the question comes back to him. It comes out that he's run for Congress, worked as a speechwriter in Washington, and is now going back to Dallas as a lawyer. He says, "I am ambitious. But it's sometimes unpleasant to be thought of as ambitious. After I got hired by this law firm I noticed there were no black people. I asked for a black secretary. It's not much, it just came up . . . An old friend of mine said to me, 'Shrewd move, Lon.' And I thought, *Goddamn, I thought he knew me.* Now, on this trip of ours I wasn't the young executive. I wasn't expected to be, and we didn't need it. So it wasn't that I was being different, it was that the situation was different in a way that I needed . . ."

It is true that one of the discoveries people can make on Outward Bound trips is the pleasant efficiency of anarchy. You may not end up converted, but you can see the possibility for a while. There is, of course, a need for competence, but competence bubbles *up* better than when it comes *down* from on high. And there is even more group response to the pieces of voluntary goodwill (giving the Reese's Peanut Butter Cup in your pocket to someone colder, getting up first to make breakfast, even just having a good time) than there is to executive rule.

So now, at the last campfire, while I list as my high points items of natural beauty, I also mention a moment late in the trip. I came back into camp dragging a small dead tree for firewood, and suddenly I saw this randomly assembled group as a little tribe—a peaceful tribe of wood gatherers, fire makers, soup brewers, igloo builders, and snowshoe menders. What would have appeared to a movie camera as leaderless, aimless fussing was order of a different order. We hadn't lived as part of nature, but we had been, in Thoreau's phrase, "sojourners in nature."

Ocean State Marathon

My friend Bill Keough wanted to run a marathon just to see if he could. He said, "You should give it a try. I've picked the Rhode Island marathon because it's flat. And it's in Newport, just across the bay from you. Come on. It'll cheer you up."

I'd won a Guggenheim Fellowship and decided to spend the year back in Rhode Island. Beware of good luck on one front. After that good news, every time the phone rang the news was bad. Even a bad dream I had turned out to be true. I'd list the bad news, but it would sound like a woe-woe-woe country-and-western song. The first line would be "After my old dog died, things just went from bad to worse. Four funerals and my own divorce."

Keough was a help. He got me to run, and he got me to laugh. We came up with a ten-week training plan. I'd been jogging about twenty miles a week and sometimes added a twenty-minute swim to a four-mile run, especially if I'd gone through some poison ivy. Saltwater sucks away the poison-ivy juice. We decided on thirty, thirty-five, forty, forty-five, fifty, fifty-five, sixty, sixty-five, seventy—and during that seventy-mile week do one run that's two-thirds of a marathon, call it eighteen miles. Then cut back to fifty and take it easy the week before. Like a good Stakhanovite, I overfulfilled the ten-week plan, adding a few miles and some swimming. I'd also heard that it was a good idea to vary the mileage and the speed.

On nine- or ten-mile runs I'd sometimes zone out, semi-hypnotized. Once in a while I'd snap out of it to find myself wondering how I got where I was. A few weeks into the plan, it felt good to go faster. I ran a 10K race in Providence, not all *that* fast but a personal best. The only unpleasant part was that after I finished I was walking back alongside the course, cheering on the later runners. A guy came trotting along, an Irish flag on his T-shirt. I yelled, "Up the Republic!" He yelled back, "Up yours, too, buddy." What? Didn't he know the first thing about Irish history? If I'd said, *"Erin go bragh"* . . . Oh, never mind.

I'd delayed registering for the marathon, and it was booked up. Luckily, a guy I met out running had registered and decided not to run Ocean State. He said I could use his name and number.

The Ocean State Marathon goes around Newport, Rhode Island, two and a half times. No hills, just some lazy, gentle slopes, crisp salt air, and a view of the "cottages"—the robber-baron piles that got Henry James steamed.

At the start elite front-runners took off; the rest of us shuffled along slowly until the crowd thinned.

Keough and I made a pact to stick together for the first twenty miles. After that, every man for himself. We loped along comfortably at about eight or nine minutes a mile. It was chilly, but I'd found a spare pair of socks in the car, and they did for mittens. The other bare parts were warm after the first two miles. After the tenth mile we stopped talking. The next hour or so was the longest time I ever spent with Keough without either of us saying a word. At mile twenty, he waved me on.

A lot of runners call mile twenty "the wall." You've used up your available blood sugar long before, and you're probably doing something terrible to your liver or kidneys. But our pace had been relatively leisurely, and I felt a crazy surge of energy. It might have been endorphins, or—and this is more likely—it might have been a bit of mania after being mournful. I'd been pretty much down every day except for the hour or so of running and an hour afterward. At mile twenty I felt wild. I felt like a lion—no, they're good only for a sprint— like a wolf. I once saw a pack of wolves from a hilltop. They streamed up the valley like a banner in the wind.

I caught up to a bunch of runners who were moving at a good pace, maybe not as fast as wolves, but I did get a boost from being in a pack.

One of the front-runners began to hobble, then limped to the side of the road and sat down. She clutched her calf. Pretty clearly a cramp. Part of euphoria is that you think it's up to you to save the world. I knelt in front of her like a shoe salesman. I said, "This'll hurt for a second, but then it'll be better." I pulled her toes up toward her knee. The calf cramp eased.

She said, "Thank you, thank you." I ran after the pack, even more euphoric after thirty seconds of a Boy Scout good deed. Well, not pure good deed. She was very pretty.

I saw the sign for mile twenty-three. I hit mile twenty-four after an overly ambitious seven-minute mile. I began to feel less fluid. I reined in a bit. I distracted myself by trying to remember how much longer than twenty-six miles a marathon is. A fifth of a mile? A quarter? To hell with it. Just run. Just be thankful that for a while you don't feel the stone of grief in your chest.

A guy passed me. I fell in behind him, picking up his rhythm. He seemed intent on catching my old wolf pack. I thought, *Oh, yeah, this is a race.* He led me past a few runners of the now-broken-up pack. When the finish line was in sight I thought it would be ungrateful of me to pass him.

And then it was over. I thought I would walk back along the course to look for Keough or the calf-cramp woman. I began to shiver and decided to go back to the car for my sweat suit. By the time I got warm clothes on, the whole thing seemed to have taken place long ago.

Intervals

fter the Ocean State Marathon I went out to San Francisco to be comforted by my middle sister and brother-in-law. My sister arranged lunches with writer friends of hers. She and Harold took me to concerts. Harold and I went running; all three of us went bicycling.

Then I went to the MacDowell Colony for two months, packing up my little pickup with a duffel bag of clothes, my typewriter, my cross-country skis, and my bicycle.

In late February and early March it didn't snow, so I jogged and bicycled. Later in March it snowed and snowed. My day was breakfast at eight-fifteen, work until lunch, take a break, work for three more hours, and then go out for an hour or more of skiing through the woods. A good thing about cross-country skiing is that you can follow your tracks back home. A good thing about artists' colonies is that you can work until you're exhausted and you don't have to keep in reserve the energy it takes to be cheerful when opening a can of Campbell's soup for one. There's a gang for supper.

After supper I'd go to the laundry room and wash my cross-country skiing clothes. While watching my clothes whirl around I'd type up what I'd written in longhand during the day. And so to bed.

I asked to stay on for another month. The director said there were no heated studio cabins. I asked if there was a fireplace. She said, "Yes, but there's no woodpile." I said that I had a small saw and an ax, and I could tell deadwood from live. She said, "Okay."

I've always liked chopping and sawing, so I added a half hour of those in the morning and went running in the late afternoon, long runs with lots of hills. I'd heard about interval training only thirdhand. I knew that cross-country skiing over rolling ground has built-in intervals. Pant hard going uphill and catch a break going down. I kept up that rhythm after the snow melted. I rented a tiny cabin near Adamsville, Rhode Island, near the head of the west branch of the Westport River. What I hadn't realized is that three months of writing double shifts, plus doing a bit of revising, which I typed in front of the washing machine, had to be paid for. I couldn't write a word in the tiny cabin for one.

I'd chosen to be in Adamsville, Rhode Island, so I could visit my daughters, whom I missed terribly.

What with the frustration of not writing and the loneliness, I would have gone nuts without rowing in the morning and running in the afternoon. I found a series of road races in Rhode Island—"Runs for Fun"—so I picked up the pace of the afternoon runs. The first couple of races I was in the middle of the pack. A kindly soul pointed out that I was starting out too slow. "You've got to be more daring." On the third one I took my daughters along, promising them supper and a movie afterward. We got to the start late, but the race administrators told me there was a shorter race around several playing fields at the University of Rhode Island. Only a mile and a quarter. It was on well-kept grass, mowed short. My daughters were much happier with that arrangement. They could sit in the baseball bleachers and watch the whole race and be off to supper much earlier. I promised them it wouldn't take long at all—ten minutes, max.

As I was warming up I noticed there was a group of ten serious runners. They were wearing spiked track shoes. I thought I'd try to hang with them for the first half, just to see what it felt like to run fast. It felt wonderful for a while. Then it felt pretty bad.

The spiked-shoe runners had friends or coaches yelling out their quarter-mile splits. I didn't pay attention at first, just concentrated on hanging with the ten fast guys. Then I heard someone shout, "Last half-mile! Get closer! Get closer if you want to make a move."

The runner in front of me was the one being yelled at. I thought, *Let's see. Let's do what the coach says. What the kind soul said. "Be more daring."*

It felt better. That was a surprise. A gift out of the air. Go with it, use it up.

We came around a curve. Now I felt pain again, but it didn't matter; it didn't matter that my guts felt as though they were burning a hole in me. I was running fast. And then another gift out of the air, a wish to use everything until there was nothing, nothing but running faster.

I have no memory of the last part of the race. I can't remember seeing anything but the green grass beyond the finish line. I remember coming back into my body, perhaps when I told myself to keep jogging, to follow the spiked-shoe runners onto the infield to get out of the way of the rest of the pack.

After all the runners finished I saw Maud and Nell climbing down the bleachers. Maud said, "Dad. Dad, you were really cooking."

A man came up to Maud and Nell and me. He said, "You're over forty, right?"

"I'm forty-one."

"Good. I'm scouting for Bill Cosby. He wants to put together an over-forty mile relay team. I think you've got quarter-mile speed. Your time for the first mile was six-thirty-one. Your last quarter was a negative split, faster than your first quarters. You came in ninth, beat one of the college boys. Here's my card. You do much interval training?"

"Some."

"Do some more, and then come to Philadelphia in a month."

I vaguely remembered that Bill Cosby had run track at Temple. Maybe it was true. I asked how old Bill Cosby was.

"About your age."

"Tell me more about intervals."

"Oh. Ten times two hundred meters. Maybe some three hundreds. A minute or so rest in between. There's books on the subject."

I lost the card. I couldn't have done it anyway. Maud and Nell had to be driven to summer camp, and I still wanted to take another stab at writing in the tiny cabin. To this day I don't know if the Bill Cosby over-forty relay team was a possibility. It did have an effect on me. I saw an ad in the newspaper for the Rhode Island Senior Olympics, to take place at the Brown University stadium three weeks after the mile-and-a-quarter Run for Fun. "Senior" meant over forty. I signed up. I bought a pair of emerald-green spiked track shoes. Once in a while it helps to buy equipment you have to live up to.

I was still frustrated by trying to write, although a few lines squirted out onto index cards. But I did take up interval training more seriously. I ran on Horseneck Beach. I didn't have a stopwatch, but I'd run for thirty seconds by the sweep hand of my wristwatch, walk a bit, and do it again. I'd end up way east, and then jog slowly back and up over the dunes to where I'd left my pickup. I did find a book, soon enough to learn that you're supposed to do speed work only every other day. Every *other* other day was LSD (long slow distance).

I showed up at the Brown stadium and felt very alone. Most of the contestants came as members of one track club or another. I signed up for the one-hundred-, the two-hundred-, and the four-hundred-meter races, as well as the shot put and the javelin. I came in second in the preliminary heat for the one hundred, came in fourth in the final, no medal, out of the hardware. The shot put was dismal. I couldn't remember how to do it.

Warming up for the four hundred, which I hadn't run in high school, I was puzzled. Was there a strategy? I'd run a practice four hundred in fifty-seven seconds. It had hurt a lot near the end. I thought I should shoot for that, which meant a 26.5 for the first two hundred meters. I gave my watch to a kid and asked him to stand at the halfway mark and tell me how many seconds. I wasn't in a normal state of mind. I'd been alone in the cabin a lot.

Of course the kid couldn't calculate by the sweep hand— I couldn't do it myself. On the beach I'd wait for the hand to hit noon and then go for my thirty-second interval. What the kid did do was cheer as I ran past him. I was third, feeling okay. Passed one guy on the backstretch, hung on the leader's tail, hoping he'd take the final turn wide. He did. I squeezed inside. That cheered me up enough to outsprint him in the last one hundred.

And there came the kid trotting across the infield with my watch. I bought him a Coke, little enough for bucking up my faith in random twelve-year-olds.

I hadn't touched a javelin since I was seventeen. At first I couldn't remember whether I'd used the Finnish back step or the Swedish front step at the end of the run-in. I did remember that I shouldn't pull my throwing arm back as I approached the line, but instead run past the javelin to cock it, so to speak. I went over the line on the first throw. I fouled on the second throw, too. *Damn.* And they weren't bad throws. A man came up to me. He said, "Put your sweatshirt beside the last bit of the run-in. Put it a yard farther back from where you started your throw this last time." I thanked him. He said, "I'm doing my third throw now. You can use my javelin. It's better than the one they gave you."

I watched him. Nifty throw. Way out there. The official put a little flag where it hit. The man brought the javelin to me. "Okay," he said. "It's my personal javelin. Get the feel of it. And watch for your mark."

I liked the feel of it. I trotted alongside the run-in with it. Put my sweatshirt down. Walked back to the start of the run-in. I thought of what I'd felt like twenty-five years before, edited out everything but my best throw. *Okay, like that.* Let muscle memory come out of the past.

One of the pleasures of throwing a javelin is that you can watch it. After putting the shot, you barely have time to turn your head and it's gone *ker-thunk* into the ground. After you throw the javelin and are hopping on one foot safely behind the foul line, you can watch the javelin fly for what seems like a long time. Even if the throw is not so hot, the javelin makes a lovely arc.

I didn't foul. I kept my balance and watched. It felt like a good throw. It looked like a good throw. I saw the flag where my new friend's throw had landed. I thought, *Oh, God, I don't want to beat him.* The javelin was coming down. For an instant it looked like it was going past the flag. And then relief. Two feet short.

I retrieved the javelin and brought it back to him. I thanked him. He said, "Good throw. Very close. For a second there, my heart was in my throat."

I said, "It worked out right."

He offered to buy me a drink. I said I had to get ready for the two hundred meters.

"You're keeping yourself busy."

"I've been sort of cooped up for a while."

He was the second person I'd talked to that day—in fact, for the last two weeks, not counting the cashier at the Adamsville General Store. I was batting two for two in the kindness-of-strangers department.

I did okay in the two-twenty (another silver), but it was the kid and the javelin thrower who made the day. The track meet got me over being a hermit. I called up some old friends in Providence, wondered why on earth I hadn't before. Even Thoreau, when he was living by Walden Pond, used to take his laundry to his mother's, maybe drop by Emerson's house.

I went up to Providence a couple of times a week.

The event that gave me the most pleasure that year came by chance. I'd done a marathon, cross-country skied a lot, run hard in the mile and a quarter, done intervals to prepare for the quarter-mile. That was enough of *that* stuff. I settled for comfortable sightseeing rows and runs. One evening I was passing a field. A farmer and two of his children were loading hay bales onto a wagon. I jogged over and asked if they could use a hand. The farmer took in my running shorts and tank top. "You ever stacked bales?"

"Yes. I used to work for a farmer in Iowa."

I knew to set the rough-cut end of one bale against the

smooth end of another. When the stack on the wagon got high, I remembered how to use a pitchfork to spear a bale and lift it, then use my right hand to shoot the shaft of the pitchfork through the loosened grip of my left hand and heave the bale up to the top of the load. It was a muscle memory as satisfying as the Finnish back step. (This is now a useless skill—no more rectangular bales.) One son was up on top, fitting the bales together. The other son was on the other side of the wagon, doing the same thing I was on mine. The farmer drove the tractor pulling the wagon, trundling along at a walking pace. We emptied wagonload after wagonload in the barn loft.

It occurred to me that lofting bales would be good weight training for javelin throwing. Then I thought I had it the wrong way around. This was the end event. It took about an hour and a half to finish the field. It was twilight.

The farmer asked me to supper, but I said I had to get home and shower, I was too sweaty to sit down at a supper table. The farmer said, "Well, then, thank you. You showed up at a good time."

I walked home, too tired to run the last couple of miles but happily, usefully, tired.

I loaned my skiff to a friend who'd built a house on Peter's Creek in South Dartmouth, Massachusetts, and said another good-bye to New England. I'd be back for the skiff one way or another.

Into the Woods
(Tom "Tracker" Brown)

I n the clearing around the lodge, fifty people are trying to start fifty fires. Each has a knife, a piece of cord, and some wood. They have been at it for some time now, and most of them have made several mistakes. There are lots of mistakes to make.

We had watched a demonstration in which the instructor had started a fire with his bow and drill in less than a minute, even going slowly and holding up the pieces of equipment one by one for us to see. These pieces are: (1) A piece of bark. (2) Tinder, but not just any old stuff. Fibers as thin as thread, fluffed up into a ball the size of a small bird's nest—so dry you have to keep it in your pocket, where it can't absorb moisture from the air. (3) The fireboard. At least a hand's length—from wrist to fingertip—a hand's breadth, and a thumb thick. Must be *flat*. (4) Drill. Hand's length and thumb thick also, but must be *round*—as round as a dowel. Pointed at either end but not like a pencil. A short, sharp taper, like a votive candle. Must be the same medium-grade wood as the board. (5) Bow. Arm's length. Curved. Any wood, so long as it won't crack. Thumb thick or more. Notched to secure. (6) The cord, which could be a shoelace or twisted plant fibers. The cord should be tied loose enough to twist once around the drill. (7) Handheld block. For a right-hander, the block must fit comfortably into the left palm, or you won't be able to bear down on it.

Assembling these items from scratch takes a while. Except for the bow, we are working with cedar. We have the luxury of several axes and hatchets to split the cedar trunks into chunks, but there is a lot of whittling to get them flat, and even more whittling to turn a chunk of cedar into a dowel. Several people try to drill with pieces that are not uniformly round. The encircling bowstring slips to the narrowest part and slides uselessly, or it hangs up on a cedar knot and binds.

If the fireboard isn't flat, it's hard to start charring in the hole straight up and down. If the drill isn't straight up and down, it keeps hopping out.

If the bowstring is loose enough to slip slightly, you create just enough heat to fire-harden the hole. The hole becomes quite beautiful, resembling a dark glaze—but then you might as well try to start a fire with glass. Scrape the hole out if you can, or adjust the bow and burn in a new hole.

A dozen people get good holes in their fireboards and hand-holds. There is a twittering and squeaking noise from these bows and drills that sounds like a flock of angry terns. But, alas, a few of these holes have been burned in too close to the edge of the fireboard and crumble out. Several others are too far from the edge, which makes cutting a notch in from the edge nearly impossible.

The notch is yet another crucial piece of precision. It is the channel by which the hot cedar dust can be made to fall out of the hole and onto the tinder, which is clamped between the fireboard and the dry piece of bark and also fluffs out from the bottom of the notch to form a receiving bed.

There are now more and more twitterings and squeakings. There is also, even in this open air, a lovely smell of charring cedar.

The first hole I burn into my fireboard is aslant and too close to the edge. Trying to start a new hole with the point of my Swiss Army Knife, I snap the blade shut and slice into the pad of my middle finger.

There are three other blood-sprinkled fireboards in the course of the morning. Someone once warned me about folding knives. It comes back to me now. It also occurs to me how hard this fire building would be with a stone knife. My admiration for our Neolithic predecessors rises.

While waiting for the blood to clot, I watch some other people getting close. One woman—very close, indeed—arranges her tinder under her fireboard notch. She lubricates the hole in the handhold with some grease from the side of her nose so that the handhold won't have enough friction to burn anymore—it's the fireboard you want to burn, not the handhold. She twists her drill into the bowstring, fits the charred end into the notched, blackened hold in the fireboard, and caps the top end of the drill with her handhold. Her left foot is already on the fireboard. She edges it closer to the drill and gets her chest down on her left knee, her left wrist held steady against the upper shin. She starts stroking smoothly and then leans into it, bearing down harder and harder, stroking furiously. Smoke begins to curl from the drill end. She is panting. More and more smoke. If she goes on any longer, the notch will clog with hot dust and go out. She stops and flicks a twig down through the notch, then scoops up the tinder and holds it in front of her mouth, puffing.

"Not so hard," one of the instructors says. Too late. She has blown it out.

Downhearted for only a minute, she fluffs up her tinder and adds some more to make up for what she's scorched.

"Just breathe on it at first. When it smokes more, blow. When you get thick smoke, blow harder. You'll get it."

The first student fire comes at mid-morning. An hour of theory, an hour and a half of whittling and fiddling. It is a doctor who fires first: good manual dexterity, as he later illustrates by stitching up a hand.

The woman who came close has shaken out the fatigue in her bowing arm and goes again. Good, thick smoke. She flicks the hot stuff out of the notch and nests it in the tinder. Kneeling, she holds up the fluff with both sets of fingertips. She looks like a priestess in an excited trance, breathing more and more rapidly. She purses her lips—four good puffs and there is a magnificent burst of flame. Applause from the crowd.

After three hours or so we go back to the lodge for the next lesson—shelter. Only a third of us have made fire. I finally get mine during a short break the next morning. It is as big a thrill as catching my first fish when I was nine. Part of the thrill is that one's individual initiation is a reenactment of an event that, replicated throughout families and tribes, changed the nature of human life.

•◆•

Who are all these people? How did they get up to this cleft in the Blue Ridge?

A lot of them are Sierra Club members who read about the course in a club bulletin. Some of them read about it in *Mother*

Earth News. Some more read a condensed version of *The Tracker* by Tom Brown Jr. in *Reader's Digest* and came for his course.

When I saw the ad in the Charlottesville *Daily Progress,* I thought a lot of these people would be survivalists—people who have stored food and water in their fallout shelters—but this isn't the case. They are all fairly adept at backpacking and camping, apparent from the neat little tents scattered around the lodge clearing. When everyone leaves late Sunday afternoon, there isn't a trace.

In fact, Tom Brown mocks the survivalists in their fortresses with a ton of canned goods. What most of the people here want for their $175—somewhat higher for those who are not Sierra Club members—is the sort of resourceful skill that would be crucial if they were lost on a hike, benighted, and caught by a sudden turn of weather—or possibly abandoned in the wilderness by a car breakdown or a plane crash.

Part of what Tom "Tracker" Brown wants for us is something like that. He says that he has taught thousands of people this course in three-day, seven-day, and longer versions, and that hundreds of people have written to him gratefully to say that they've had to use these skills. But there is more to it than that. Even though he outlines what he has in mind during the first session on Friday night, the import of it doesn't begin to come clear until later. To some extent, what Tom Brown has to say can't be said.

The flavor of the man also takes some getting used to. It certainly had a push-pull effect on me at first: resistance and fascination.

Tom Brown's first appearance is commanding. He's a bit over six feet tall, with thick shoulders and upper arms but with a well-centered ease of movement. He has light, almost shoulder-length hair and blue eyes with hazel flecks. The eyes are close together and intense.

Early Friday evening, he said, "On your way to the lodge, did you see the moon? Is it full? Where is it? Did you notice the wind shifts? Were you aware of the frogs? The ten different frogs? Did you hear the birds? The forty bird voices? Right here outside the lodge, did you see the weasel? The fox? The deer? The red squirrel? Yes, the red squirrel is nocturnal. Did you see the mouse behind me here?"

He took a breath and then went into a rant that started piano but ended fortissimo. "I see by the fancy binoculars that some of you are carrying that we have some bird-watchers. Okay, fine. But here's what some birders are like . . . One time I was on a cruise boat in the Everglades, and I heard a woman say to the man next to her, 'What's that huge bird?' The man said, 'Oh, that. That's only a vulture.' I turned around and grabbed the lapels of his jacket. I said, *'Only a vulture*! Have you climbed up to look in a vulture's nest and *had one puke in your face?* That's what a vulture does. When you've had one puke in your face, *then* you can say *"Only a vulture."*'"

That was the most alarmingly intense part of the hour-long lecture. Everyone, Tom Brown included, took a deep breath. He went back to outlining the practical skills he and his staff would be teaching us.

Tom Brown is a tracker. He's been called in by the police to find criminals and missing persons. But he's not going to talk about that, except to say that he's seen survival situations of both kinds. Both kinds? "I've pulled the frozen bodies out of survival situations that didn't work."

He is going to teach us four basic survival skills. The big three are: (1) How to find and make shelter. "You can survive naked at forty below with a shelter you can make with your

bare hands." (2) How to find water. (3) How to make fire without manufactured aid. We are allowed to use knives on this
trip, but we learn how to fracture rocks to get a sharp-edged
tool.

The fourth survival skill is how to find food. "Any one of
you here could survive for twenty days without food. I've gone
without food for forty days and not been debilitated. I just lost
twenty pounds," he says.

We took up fire making bright and early Saturday morning because it's the most physically difficult. Now we're back
inside the lodge after a quick lunch of stew from the twenty-
gallon cauldron over the communal campfire. A slide show
of shelters—wickiups, wigwams, tepees, hogans—ends with
step-by-step directions for the Tom Brown special, the debris
hut, good to forty below. This is something I know a little bit
about, having spent several days alone in a snow cave of my
own construction.

As with almost all of the techniques we learned from Tom,
this shelter had an animal slogan. "How do you build a shelter? Go ask the squirrel." This style of instruction was something he had learned from his mentor, an old Apache. Tom
met Stalking Wolf when Tom was eight years old, Stalking
Wolf eighty-three. He spent his spare time from eight to sixteen with Stalking Wolf and his grandson, who was the same
age as Tom. If you listen to this style with a cynical ear, it
can sound like *Tarzan* comic-book bubbles. Simba the lion,
Tantor the elephant. "Taste the bite of my steel tooth," Tarzan
exclaims as he swings down on a charging warthog.

But all good ideas have their burlesque possibilities. The
particularity and accuracy of the Stalking Wolf proposi-
tions make them attractive, rather like tai chi's mnemonics,
little crystals of appreciation for animals. What is addition-

ally attractive is that the instructive animals in Tom's primer are everyday ones, such as mice, squirrels, and chickadees—Stalking Wolf's favorite.

The debris hut is a squirrel's nest rigged on the simplest frame. We built one at a leisurely pace. A single person might have to spend an hour or two once a good spot is found. The design is simple. Prop a ridgepole against a rock or a tree notch—the notch should be three feet high, maximum. Anchor the foot of the pole on the ground and run ribs from the ridgepole to the ground. Keep the interior space only slightly larger than body size. Pile leaves, ferns, pine needles, moss, twigs—anything—on the ribs. Keep the pile in place with interlaced vines and sticks. Pile on more debris, more vines and sticks. Keep the general shape slanted so rain will run off. Add more debris until you can sink your whole arm into it: the debris doesn't have to be dry—just thick. Crawl in and look for light coming through chinks. Crawl out and cover them. Then fill the interior with debris. Crawl in. Crawl out. Fill the hole you make with more debris. Crawl in, crawl out. Add more debris. Make a bundle of leaves and bind it together with vines, grasses, or flexible twigs—or, for the more advanced, weave a basket and fill it with leaves. Crawl in and plug the entrance behind you with the bundle of debris.

I crawled into the shelter we'd built. It was dark—good, no chinks—and noisy from the rustling leaves. After a while, I could feel my trapped body heat. To be sure, this was a pleasant, dry fall day, but the leaves felt as surprisingly cozy as a goose-down coat. I should not have been surprised. The shelter works on the same trapped-air principle as insulated coats and sleeping bags, and what we'd done with our clumps of leaves and sticks was to make a giant sleeping bag with four feet of "loft" rather than four inches.

•◆•

Back at the lodge to learn about water. Of the big three survival skills, finding water is the easiest, according to Tom. As there was a lake practically at our elbow, this proposition didn't seem unlikely.

We learned about solar stills, getting water from trees and plants—you can get water from a wild grapevine by clipping a runner near the bottom and letting the liquid flow down into your cup. You can even get it from as simple but plentiful a method as sponging up dew with a T-shirt.

The main problem with water in America isn't finding it, it's getting rid of the pollution. More and more, previously safe streams and groundwater have dangerous organisms. Most of these can be killed by a ten-minute boil—up from the five-minute boil suggested in most survival manuals: the bacteria are getting hardier. But there's not much that can be done about chemical pollutants. Even sand and charcoal filters don't work.

This is depressing to contemplate. But it was somewhere around this stage of the weekend that I felt either a change in the instruction or, possibly, more at ease myself. One of the surprises about Tom Brown's instructions is that there is no separation between the "go ask the squirrel" mode and his summarizing the latest report from a university testing laboratory. Like many bright, largely self-taught people, Tom Brown has an occasionally contemptuous attitude toward, say, Ph.D.s or lawyers. But this is not a rejection of logic or science.

Later in the evening—after water, deadfalls and snares, and

edible plants—when we are sitting around in small groups, making cordage out of fibers, Tom mentions that pokeweed looks as if it has some cancer-inhibiting qualities. I'd heard a lot of this talk about miraculous nuts and berries during the *Whole Earth Catalog* days, not to mention the later Laetrile stories.

I say a little wryly to the oncologist who is braiding his rope beside me, "Use much pokeweed these days?"

He says, "Not yet. We're still testing it on animals. It looks promising."

But it isn't the confirmation from my own off-and-on camping experience or this spot-check scientific validation that warms me up. It is a combination of a great many things that begin to fit together in a coherent picture. There is a romantic and a horrific side—for example, Tom Brown's story about tracking a deer, lying in wait in a tree above its run, dropping on it, missing the clean kill because his knife handle broke, and having to strangle it, an avowedly painful process. He says that at last "I felt the deer's spirit slip through my fingers." When Tom told Stalking Wolf about it—so Tom must have been sixteen or younger—Stalking Wolf said, "When you can feel that spirit in a blade of grass, then you will be one with nature."

This narrative gives me some trouble. I finally realize that it is more my own discomfort, the incoherence of my own attitudes toward nature as well as my literary preference for understatement and indirection. One can even suspect that Tom Brown is telling the story in part for the shock value and still be grateful for the confrontation with one's own killing for meat, even if only by the agency of slaughterhouses. It reminded me of rabbit, quail, pheasant, turtle, fish, and shellfish of several kinds that I'd killed and eaten—some with attentiveness, and some not.

By now there are several clues that whatever strong, macho scent of the man I might have sniffed initially, there is another savor of attentiveness, enthusiasm, and marveling tenderness. I am reminded of the man who taught me how to fish for striped bass. After he'd taught me some of the where and how, he took me out one night when there were a good many phosphorescent plankton in the water. We hung over the gunwale and simply watched the flashes of light in a couple of fathoms of saltwater. Every time a fish moved at speed, it left a brief comet's trail. Dashes and swirls flared as fish fed or ran for cover. A globe of light came where a big fish fanned its tail. Some time later I saw a bar of light—probably a striper—grab a flicker of light that might have been an eel, and there was an explosion of phosphorescence.

My mentor said, "That's what goes on down there. You ought to have some notion of what you're getting into. Aside from just killing a few of them."

It was, of course, a much longer story. What striped bass eat; where what they eat comes from; what they, in turn, eat. Even just a little watching of a single fish stirs the larger web out to its invisible edges.

As I traced through what Tom Brown had been saying, I realized that very little of his time outdoors is spent in anything like blood sport. It is looking, inferring, and connecting what he sees going on. His ideal is "gentle wandering."

•◆•

Saturday was hard to take in. It consisted pretty much of uninterrupted alternations of lecture and outdoor practice from eight a.m. until past eleven p.m.: fire, shelter, water, deadfalls, snares, throwing sticks, edible plants, cordage, and tanning, which we in the short course didn't practice.

Sunday was shorter—eight a.m. to four p.m.—but in a way it was more bountiful. We took another quick shot at fire, or whatever we hadn't achieved the day before, and then spent some time learning to look and listen, which sounds dumb. But it turned out to be the most ingenious and mysterious suggestion of all.

We'd heard a little sermon Friday night about dulling habits, narrowed attentiveness. I thought it might be a case of preaching to the converted. But the more concrete explanation Sunday was amazing. Most people focus most of the time. Animals don't. So the first effort is to see more by unfocusing, then focusing on whatever seems of interest. Unfocus again. Hold your arms straight out to the sides. Try to see the fingers of both hands. Keep this breadth of vision—this unfocused vision—and move slowly through the woods. In just a short while, you'll begin to notice more.

Even this slight modification of habit was startling and, for a brief while, alarming. It felt as though protective parts of my skull were missing.

We were told that this unfocused vision is probably less tiring than the uninterrupted darting focusing that most people use most of the time.

It must have been an odd sight—fifty people fanning out from the lodge, their arms stretched wide and fingers wiggling, moving like sleepwalkers, but it was odder yet to see the stalking walk.

"Go ask the heron" was the motto for this one. This exercise would clearly take a good deal of "dirt time"—meaning fieldwork, or on-the-job training. The one immediate realization was that all those Indians in literature, from James Fenimore Cooper's to Zane Grey's, actually could have moved noiselessly. We did learn how to step on a leaf or a twig without making it crackle. It's a matter of rolling the unweighted foot sideways, then backward, then forward, then letting the weight flow forward through the hips and onto the foot that is resting on the gradually and softly flattened leaf. But it's easier said than done, and next to impossible in hiking boots. Tom and the staff wear moccasins or thin running shoes.

Tracking is the most complex subject we undertake. The hour of lecture is chock-full, even though Tom has it well broken up. "I'm not going to teach you the details you can get from *Peterson's Field Guide to Animal Tracks*. I'm going to give you the basics you can hang that on. And enough so that you can improve if you spend some dirt time."

We get an outline of the most common prints, and another outline telling which animals walk diagonally, which ones pace, which bound, which gallop. We learn how to tell a buck from a doe by the straddle of the hoofprints.

We go down to a mudflat by the lake. The mud is a *Reader's Digest* of what went on the night before: huge heron tracks, beaver, dog, deer. A few of us are able to pick up the trail of a deer leaving the lake and follow it back into the woods. I find myself standing amazed at this profusion, but it turns out there are even more tracks than the fraction I notice.

More instruction on signs. The basic technique here is to have some idea of the way everything usually is and then to notice what's different. In Tom Brown's book *The Tracker*—the first volume of his autobiography—there is his account of his tracking a retarded man who'd been missing for a couple of days. The police had given up. Tom Brown found him. The account is like a Sherlock Holmes story, but the number of deductions is squared or cubed. It's not done by eyesight alone but by a delicate touching with the pads of the fingers. A good deal of time is spent on hands and knees, squinting along the ground against the light to pick up the slightest bas-relief.

The faintest glimmer of how satisfying an art this might be, of the sort of ramifying awareness it might lead to, comes during the last dirt-time period. We've learned that the most active part of the outdoors is neither the deep forest nor the open field but the brushy transition areas near both food and cover. We string out along what could be any roadside tangle, the sort of matted grass and weeds one passes even near city vacant lots. Following Tom's suggestions, I pick the grass apart and peer down. After only a little probing, I find a vole run. The vole is a squat little thing—"the Volkswagen of rodents"—and is prey to almost everything bigger than it, and even to shrews, which are smaller. The clear network of worn paths—tunnels, really—arched over by the tangle is astounding. Tracing along this delicate labyrinth, I come on some vole scat—tiny enough to pass through the eye of a darning needle but a perfect segmented turd, perfect in a way that suddenly brings my eye into the scale of vole life, the miniature grooves of its runs through the vast forest of grass blades in which it lives.

I wander over toward Tom with this find on my fingertip to get some pointers on guessing the age of the scat. Tom is off with two of the teenagers who are taking the course. He is the most relaxed I've seen him. The reason may be, in part, that this session is almost over. He and his instructors have been going practically nonstop all weekend. But from the attitude of this trio, it's more likely he's at ease because this is the part he likes best: he's listening to the two boys, who have found a print and have figured out it's a fox. Good. Now what's the next step? They measure a fox stride and find a partial print. Good. Now what? They guess, rightly, that the fox jumped over the little gully, and they begin to hover over the ground at nose length, looking for another print.

•◆•

When I talked to Tom for a half hour earlier in the day he was less pleased with most of the group. He wasn't unhappy with our accomplishment but with what he took to be our holding back. He wants people taking his course to get into it completely.

I said that maybe some of us were taken aback by how much he was top dog, even with his group of instructors. This remark, like the rest of my questions and comments, didn't irritate him, nor did he even feel the need to present a defense. I asked some of the instructors about Tom's being the alpha dog, and they knew what I meant, but they, too, didn't think it needed explaining. It seemed perfectly natural to them in light of what they were all trying to do for us in a short time.

I ask Tom what he thinks of Outward Bound. He says that it's good at what it does, but what it does isn't what he's after. I suggest that there is at least some common ground. He listens to what I have to say. Then he mentions that several of the Outward Bound instructors have come to him to take his course. Okay. I understand that he doesn't wish to be measured by that stick.

On reflection, I can see why he doesn't. Tom, though he is an educator, is not part of the human potential movement—at least not in the sense that he wants an experience of nature to be a means to the end of a better person. Nature is the end: nature is Tom's religion. If you become more aware of nature, you'll be a better person, but the splendor is nature, not you.

It is also true that Outward Bound courses are not how-to. You do pick up a little rock climbing, some survival techniques, and other skills, but the course is designed to leave you with a sense of accomplishment. The accomplishment is to be continued, to be sure, but it is also to be savored then and there.

Tom's courses are hard-core how-to. The thrills of accomplishment are, for the most part, prospective. You get them after more dirt time, when you go off on your own. And even then, awareness, at the standard Tom sets, will be beyond what most people will attain.

I ask Tom whom he admires, apart from Stalking Wolf. It's a short list: Thoreau; John Muir—"He's a romanticist, but his early life is admirable"; Robert Bateman, a wildlife artist; and Roger Tory Peterson, who in turn admires Tom Brown. That's the standard he sets for himself—complete dedication.

And yet, to return to the final hour of the course, there is Tom, clearly enjoying enormously those two boys finding and figuring out a couple of fox prints. There is Tom, responding with enthusiasm to the perfect little vole scat I present to him on the tip of my finger. And there is the Tom Brown who, when he finally tracks down the retarded man, amid the clatter of the helicopter he's radioed in and the squad of troopers it disgorges, realizes that he is the one who knows the lost man best, and he hugs him as the man bursts into tears from fear and relief.

·◆·

We heard many more details of plant and animal lore and Native American technology than I've recorded here. These stick pleasantly to my thoughts as I walk around my home landscape, burrs and hitchhikers on the cuffs of my attention.

Tom Brown, the man, is worth the trip, too.

But what I'm happiest about in a way is the prod to my historical imagination. The parts of history most easily accessible to us are, naturally, those more fully recorded. But once in a while I've read something that made me think I was neglecting the prehistoric, or, more accurately, unchronicled history. One doesn't have to reject modern life to be moved by what we've lost, or at least misplaced, from the Neolithic heritage. Native Americans, who came to this continent during the Neolithic age, preserved a great deal of it. Tom Brown, by an odd piece of luck in his childhood, got hold of a thread leading into it, and has followed it on his own terms actively and intelligently. All the course's survival techniques—how to get out of the woods alive—while potentially useful and compellingly ingenious, aren't as important as the suggestions about how to get into the woods.

Peter's Creek to Westport Point

Westport Point, Massachusetts, is a heavenly spot with only a few bits of purgatory here and there. After Fox Island was sold, I went there to visit my old friend Duncan Kennedy and his family, all of whom had spent time on the island. The two branches of the Westport River run into each other to form Westport Harbor. Just outside the channel from the harbor to the sea, Horseneck Beach runs for miles. A short way up one branch of the Westport River there is a large salt marsh with a maze of salt creeks.

During one of my stays on Westport Point (sometimes a month in one rented cottage or another, sometimes living communally with the Kennedys), I remembered that I'd loaned my old Cape Dory 16 (actually not a dory but a fiberglass version of a Whitehall skiff) to a friend who'd built her own house on a little creek near South Dartmouth. I bicycled over to see if the boat was still there. Paula wasn't home, but I found the skiff. The wooden gunwales looked okay. The plug still fit tight in the drain. The oars were okay. I slid her into Peter's Creek just to check her out. The creek level was too low to row properly, so I drifted to find a deeper bit. By the time I got to where the creek joins the Slocum River, I saw that the tide was going out too fast to get back. In my mind's eye

I tried to see a map. In two or three miles I'd get to the sea. Maybe eight miles to Gooseberry Neck. The neck juts pretty far out, and there's often rough water at the tip, but the base is narrow. I could haul the boat across. Then an unknown number of miles to Westport Harbor. I remembered from an old map that there was a public right-of-way near the very end of Westport Point.

I rowed briskly down the river, happy to have chanced into more exercise than a bike ride.

After a pleasant mile or so the screws holding the piece of wood in which the starboard oarlock was set began to wobble. I pulled to shore, thanked whichever uncle had told me always to carry a Swiss Army Knife, and cut a twig. I jammed the twig into the screw holes and reset the screws. Close enough for government work.

I rowed until I heard the sound of surf. I hadn't thought of surf. I shipped the oars and stood up to take a look. Far to one side of the now very broad river, the current had cut a channel. It was deep enough so that there was no shallow bottom to trip the waves into breaking. There was a bouncy chop where the outgoing current hit the incoming waves, but the skiff rode through it nicely. The ebb gave her a surprisingly long ride out to sea.

There was a fair-sized swell, but the spacing between crest and trough was so wide that even taking them on the beam wasn't a problem. It was like cross-country skiing across gently rolling ground—a bit harder up and then a bit easier down.

From the crests I could see Cuttyhunk, the southernmost of the Elizabeth Islands, and after a while I could see Gay Head, the high cliff at the western end of Martha's Vineyard.

When I turned to look past the bow I saw the sun lowering. As I rowed and looked astern I saw the moon rise. There wasn't another boat in sight. At first the aloneness was pleasant. Then I had a moment of worrying, not about anything in particular at first. Then about the oarlock—what if it worked loose again? I should have cut some spare twigs. Then about a sudden change in the weather. Then about what my sixteen-foot white boat might look like to a like-sized white shark.

But then this little turbulence of worries vanished into the twilight.

The wake off the stern was a reassuring sign of progress; the lift and slide of the swells made the skiff feel as if she was, in a phrase from long-ago reading, "cradled on the bosom of the deep." That rhythm helped my own, got me to relax on the recovery and pull hard on the stroke.

The sun had set; the moon had risen higher. The stars came out. It was glorious.

There wasn't enough light to read my watch. It was summer, so sunset must have been . . . eight? nine? It finally occurred to me that my wife and the Kennedys might be wondering where I was.

I sped up some, and at last I saw Gooseberry Neck, a long darkness across the not-so-dark water and against the starry sky.

I was out fairly far, so I headed in to get to the base of the neck. I saw a single small point of light. I rowed toward it, coasted ashore on a wave. The light came from a trailer. I was surprised. There was a trailer park on the other side of Gooseberry Neck, but I'd thought these woods and this beach were part of a conservation easement.

There was a man sitting in a lawn chair. He wasn't at all alarmed. I said hello; he took a puff on his cigar and said, "Out kinda late, aren't you?"

I narrated. He nodded. I asked how far it was to Westport

Point. He said, "You got folks waiting for you there? You want to make a phone call?"

"You've got a phone out here?"

"Yes. But don't go mentioning it; I like to keep my hookup arrangements informal."

I called, relayed the directions to Duncan, who fortunately knew the back roads. He said he'd pick me up. I had a pleasant twenty-minute chat with the man in the lawn chair. He said he'd keep an eye on the boat overnight.

My second wife wasn't nearly as cross as she had a right to be. The next day she even helped Duncan and me carry the boat across the neck.

It was only another few miles to the harbor and less than a mile to Westport Point. I nosed up to a pair of docks that seemed to me to be where the public landing was.

A man strolled across the lawn and asked what I was doing. I said I thought there was a right-of-way somewhere near here.

He thought for a while. Then he said, "Technically, there is. And it's here. But nobody knows about it. You must have found an old map."

"Yes. But I won't spread it around. I'd be grateful if I could carry my skiff out to the road."

"How do you come to be here?"

I narrated, leaving out the man in the lawn chair.

"Huh. All the way from the head of the Slocum River. You can tie her up here. You want a cup of coffee?"

For several summers, until Captain Billy Tongue moved to Alaska, I kept the skiff at his dock. We had a cup of coffee if I went for a morning row, a beer if I'd been out in the afternoon. The table in his backyard was the vertebra of a whale that he'd pulled up in his trawl.

The first summer or two I was writing about a lobsterman.

I would ask Billy if something I'd written was plausible. Most often he'd say, "Oh, yeah," and offer several variations from his own experience.

I'm grateful for the free dock space but mostly for the conversations, which I remember to this day. He told me about getting driven onto a shoal near Nantucket in a storm. The seas were running high and steep, breaking onto the foredeck, working the planks apart, filling up the hold. Billy told his crew to prepare to abandon ship. The cook, who'd just been hired, didn't have a survival suit. Billy said, "The poor guy ran around offering everything he had if someone would sell him theirs."

I said, "My God. I'm trying to imagine how he felt."

Billy said, "He felt underdressed for the occasion."

As it happened, a seventh wave came along and lifted the ship clear of the shoal, the pumps worked, and she got home.

One afternoon I got in my skiff. Billy came down to see me off. There was a fresh breeze. I kept getting blown back against the dock. I caught an oar blade under it. I couldn't figure out what to do with the free oar. I backed, then rowed. I finally got the stuck oar free but got wedged sideways between docks. All this flailing took a very short time. Billy said, "Maybe you'd rather I didn't watch."

Southerners, like the Irish, are good at voluminous story-telling, but for the one-sentence dry remark, it's the Yankees.

On the other hand, Billy Tongue is a good captain and a generous man. He made time for anyone who seriously wanted to know what he knew. He was too wry to go in for the high romance of the sea, nothing like "I must go down to the seas again, to the lonely sea and the sky, / And all I ask is a tall ship and a star to steer her by." But when we were sitting around the whale vertebra and he was answering a technical question, once in a while he'd stop and say how amazed he still was by the life *in* the sea, by how much was going on down there that he got only hints of.

I got a lot of instruction and, even better, a sense of his life at sea.

All that came my way from getting in my skiff and accidentally rowing from Peter's Creek to Westport Point.

Fiftieth Birthday, January 18, 1989

In January my wife was away painting. I was at home with five-year-old Clare. Maud and Nell were in college. I got an overnight babysitter so I could walk fifty kilometers from midnight to eight a.m. My third sister, an astrologer, assured me that eight a.m. was my birth hour.

My wife called from her artists' colony to make sure I was dressing Clare warmly enough. I mentioned my birthday plan. She was okay with the babysitter part but said, "You may not go by yourself. What if you sprain your ankle? What if you run into a bear?"

"It's January. Bears hibernate." But why spoil her time painting? I'd already worried her enough by going down the James alone in a canoe and rowing out to sea at night.

Luckily, I had an MFA student who'd spent the previous year trekking in Nepal. Leigh and I got dropped off at midnight in the Blue Ridge Mountains, at a spot fifty kilometers from my house. We would follow the ridge for a long bit, then saunter downhill from a gap. The last bit was on two-lane blacktop, which I thought would have little traffic at six a.m. On the drive up we left a quart of water and two chocolate bars by a signpost. We drank a lot of water so we wouldn't have to carry anything but a small canteen.

It wasn't a major effort or much of an adventure—just something to start the year off. I thought I would have preferred the uneasiness of being alone on a winter's night, but Leigh was a pleasant surprise. To begin with, she set a brisk pace. She's a small woman, but like Tigger, "Whatever [her] weight in pounds, shillings or ounces, [she] always seemed bigger because of her bounces." She also wanted to get on with it. We'd drunk so much water, we had to urinate often during the first ten kilometers. She went into the woods to the right, I to the left. Although she was wearing long pants and a belt, she was always back on the march before I was.

The first part was up and down, which is less tiring than either steady up or steady down, as we discovered when we got to the long down. I'd wrongly imagined "saunter." We weren't at all winded, but we both had tired legs by the time we got to the signpost with the water bottle and chocolate bars. The other wrongly imagined part was that there wouldn't be traffic on the two-lane blacktop at six a.m. The ridge had been still winter air, glimpses of stars, noises in the woods. (An odd note: there is a hyper-amplification of noise: a squirrel hopping in dry leaves sounds like a raccoon; a raccoon sounds like a large dog. If there'd actually been a dog, we would have thought we'd roused a bear.) Now there were frequent whooshing pickup trucks, mostly headed into town, but the few coming toward us blinded us with their high beams. Both to revive our tired legs and to get this part over quicker, we decided to jog. With only four miles to go, we took a detour on the fairway of a golf course. The very last part was on sidewalks, like walking home from work. I was suddenly tired, more from staying up all night than anything else. Leigh had wisely taken a nap the afternoon before. The last half-mile uphill, she was elated—I was sleepwalking.

I checked on Clare and the babysitter, both still asleep. I asked Leigh if she'd like breakfast. Leigh laughed. "You're out on your feet. Is the babysitter taking care of Clare for the rest of the morning?" I had to think for a slow ten seconds. "Yes. Drive her to kindergarten. Soon."

Leigh led me upstairs, turned down the covers. I sank into bed with my clothes on. Leigh took off my boots and tucked me in. She said, "I'd better come pick you up for your afternoon class. I'll come early enough so you can eat."

"Yes. Eat."

She said, "That was fun." I woke up a bit more when she touched my cheek. She said, "Happy birthday," and kissed me. It was a reverse fairy-tale kiss. It sent me into a deep sleep.

Cross-Country Skiing
with Harold in Sweden

Ten years after the very bad year, 1979, there came a wonderful year. Aside from celebrating my half-century birthday with the fifty-kilometer nightlong walk, and taking up competitive rowing again, there were other heartening events. Some publications after a drought, some prizes, though my National Book Award was immediately eclipsed by my brother-in-law, Harold Varmus, married to my middle sister. He won the Nobel Prize in Physiology of Medicine for his work on retroviruses. (That family good news was topped by my wife's announcement that she was pregnant.) I'm very fond of Harold, so without having to exercise any virtue, I rejoiced in his good fortune. I'd spent some time hiking and bicycling with him. He's one of a number of friends who is in better shape than I am. Nobel Prize winners get to bring twelve guests to Stockholm, and he included me, in part as a companion for his exercising.

"Cross-country skiing," he announced the first day. "At sunrise." I was glad we were in Sweden in December. Sunrise is about ten a.m.

He's in better shape, but at that time my technique was just enough better so we were happily matched. We skied for a couple of hours outside Stockholm. There were several circuits of trails and a lodge with saunas. It was a dream landscape of stands of evergreens and birch trees and some open fields. We got back to the lodge, turned in our rental skis, and got in a sauna. After we were roasted medium rare, I saw there was a back door. I opened it and saw a path down to a pond. There was a hole cut in the foot-thick ice. Harold said, "I'm game."

Naked as jaybirds, we walked toward the pond. A woman wearing nothing but clogs came up the path. As she came near she looked us over, said something in Swedish, and strolled on. A fleeting suspicion crossed my mind. Could she have been commenting on the effect of freezing air on naked men's bodies?

We didn't dwell on that thought, more intent on the bit of will we'd need to jump through the hole in the ice.

It was surprisingly pleasant. There was a shock of cold, but it was offset by how hot our bodies were from the sauna. We didn't linger, however. As we trotted back up the path, I felt a rush of warmth. I think my body was saying, "Help! Send hot blood to every capillary."

More sauna, a shower, and into our changes of clothes. In the lobby of the lodge we saw the Swedish woman. She said in English, "Oh. You're Americans. I thought you were Swedes. Who else jumps into freezing water?"

I said, "We were wondering what you said to us."

"I warned you that you should wear sandals or you will cut your feet on the ice."

• ◆ •

The next time we went it was with a larger group. Word had got out that a Nobel laureate was a cross-country skiing enthusiast, and the Swedes were apparently pleased that an American scientist liked their national sport. A reporter and a photographer showed up.

My old teacher Kurt Vonnegut told me that to flatter a person it's more effective to praise their minor secret vanities than their major accomplishments. (Kurt was very proud of his swimming.)

The next day Harold appeared on the front page of a Stockholm paper. The photographer had taken many pictures of Harold in graceful full stride, but the newspaper chose to run a sequence of three quick shots: Harold teetering, Harold with one ski in the air, and Harold on his ass in the snow.

When discussing science or literature Harold is serene; he even takes contradiction calmly. (See his book *The Art and Politics of Science*.) But this sharp poke at a minor vanity riled him. He was laughing but with notes of outrage.

This happened again when he was appointed head of the National Institutes of Health. An NPR reporter asked him for an interview. Harold said that every minute of his day was booked, except for the fifteen-mile bicycle ride from his house to NIH. The reporter said, "I have a bike. I'll go along, and we can do the interview as we ride."

The reporter, severely out of breath, managed to get his questions out only at traffic lights or stop signs. Harold, panting more lightly, answered. When the interview aired, the reporter's questions came out in well-modulated sentences, Harold's answers in shorter phrases, punctuated by a few quick breaths. Harold was irked again. "That . . . reporter went back and rerecorded his questions! He made it sound as if he's in better shape." Harold was laughing but with harmonics of irritation.

I'm completely sympathetic. I've had a minor vanity or two poked, once with a meta-poke. I was explaining to a class the Kurt Vonnegut theory that praising a minor vanity worked like a charm, as good a juju as a voodoo priest gathering hair clippings to cast a spell. A very bright and, what made it a bit worse, beautiful woman said, "That wouldn't work on you, John. None of your vanities are either secret *or* minor."

Our next Stockholm exercise event was an after-dark fast-paced long run. I've never been colder or more out of breath.

Very early the next morning Harold played squash. I stayed in bed until the sun rose. I didn't want to be stiff for the grand ball.

Faster Boats

I was once eating at a table full of classical scholars who were discussing *The Odyssey* and the many commentaries on it. One of them said, "My students sometimes ask me if the sea really is 'wine-dark.' I tell them the wine part is just some translator's idea. It's just dark . . . *oinos ponton*."

I couldn't help blurting, "No, wine-dark is good. Day or night, the sea is lots of colors. James Joyce has a guy call it 'snotgreen,' and that's right, too. Coincidentally, that's in *Ulysses*. But it might help to take a look. Maybe more than one look. Get hold of a rowboat and spend a couple of days at sea. As good as another commentary."

As soon as I'd blurted, I regretted it. And I *did* have a question that one of the classical scholars might have answered. I wanted to confirm something I'd heard—that the Greeks used a prototype of the sliding seat, that the Greek galley rowers sat on a piece of leather soaked in olive oil and pushed with their legs against a footrest, adding a foot or more to the length of their stroke. That would explain why the Greeks rowed circles around the Persians. I'm still looking for a classical scholar who is also a sculler. I'll approach her or him more delicately.

Modern competitive rowing developed on the Thames, among watermen who ferried passengers across and up and down the river. They raced in fixed-seat rowboats. The winners were usually long-backed, with heavily muscled arms and shoulders. The modern sliding seat was invented in the mid-nineteenth century and was in common use by 1875. The oarsmen, and eventually oarswomen, were more likely to be long-legged, with strong quadriceps, since the legs deliver about three-fourths of the drive. The swing of the back and the arm-pull provide the other quarter.

Racing crews still do pull-ups and bench pulls, but the off-the-water training has a lot of running up hills and squat lifts for leg strength.

One day while out in my Whitehall skiff, I saw an Alden ocean shell, a more stable version of a racing single shell but with a sliding seat. The rower knew how to move the boat. I'd rowed in a coxed four thirty years before, so I could appreciate the coordination of legs, back, and arms. But mainly the *Wind in the Willows* Water Rat in me went wide-eyed. I wanted one of those. I wanted to do that again, to feel what that felt like by myself. I tried out a couple of versions and settled on a modest eighteen-foot wherry with a sliding seat and old-fashioned wooden oars with soon-to-be-outmoded spoon blades. Even with a beam of about two feet, she felt very tippy. The designer of the boat, from whom I bought a demo, watched me row for a bit. He said, "If I were you, I'd take it very carefully." I rowed this wherry for a couple of years—up and down both branches of the Westport River (aka Acoaxet) and through the maze of salt creeks, getting a bit better at it. I cartopped her back to Charlottesville, wondering where I'd row. I carried her around on my car for a few days, in case I saw a likely body of water.

There was a knock on my office door, and in came a remarkably fit and beautiful woman. She said, "Would you like to be the faculty adviser to the university rowing club? You can keep your wherry in our boathouse." I must have said yes, because she said, "I'll show you where it is."

The south fork of the Rivanna has a dam, which makes a reservoir for the city of Charlottesville. Below the dam the Rivanna is a stream, but it picks up water from tributaries and is a good-sized river again by the time it joins the James. Above the dam there are five miles of almost still water. There are few houses, a couple of barns. Three miles upstream of the boathouse there's a cow pasture. Among the things to watch out for when sculling on the Rivanna are the cows that wade in and stand well out in the channel, complacently certain that the rower will avoid them. I'd never fully appreciated the weight of the word *bovine* until I turned around and looked into the untroubled eyes of a half-submerged cow. The Canada geese make way, the beavers give a startling smack with their flat tails and dive, but the cows don't even moo. I came to admire them. And learned to keep to the middle of the river.

I also saw great blue herons, wood ducks, hawks, kingfishers, grebes—and the long Rivanna Reservoir itself reflecting the blue sky and green trees. It was on their account that I inadvertently came to do interval training in a boat. I'd see the cows posing for a Flemish landscape painting, and I'd stop to admire them for a minute. Then, wanting to get in a full tour of the reservoir, I'd go hard for five or ten minutes until I'd stop to take in a great blue heron stalking minnows. Then a row of turtles basking on a log. And so on.

Occasionally there'd be a couple of eights gaining on me, and I'd speed up to get through a narrow passage before all three boats were squeezed oar blade to oar blade. One day the men's coach was out in his single. He was coming up fast, but I thought I could get through the narrows before him. For the first time I heard the higher pitch of my wake as the wherry got to her top hull speed.

When we got to the dock, the coach said, "It's a shame you didn't row in college, John."

It was a compliment, but it had a bit of the Iowa farmer seeing jogging as energy gone to waste. I said, defensively, "Well, I'm having fun now."

"Yeah, fun. But you really didn't want to get passed. Even in that bathtub you're rowing, you were racing. You should try a faster boat. There are masters' races. *Masters* means old guys."

A while later he introduced me to a visiting sculler who'd pulled up to the dock. The coach said to the sculler, "I hear you're trading up to an Empacher. You find a buyer for this one yet?"

Done and done. The only hitch was that the sculler was taking his boat to Washington to race her one last time. I was going there with an over-fifty masters' four, so that looked like it would work. But when it came time to go, two of the old guys dropped out. The coach said, "That's okay. I've got two eights and a four going, but the four only has three guys. You game?"

Our college crew came in the middle of the pack, but we did pass a Naval Academy four in the last mile. When we got to the dock, our stroke couldn't keep from saying to them, "And we had a really old professor in our boat." The coach suggested that he button it.

But the unmixed pleasure of the day was that I got my secondhand but bright-red Van Dusen. I cartopped her back to Charlottesville and took her out, twenty-seven feet long, only a couple of inches wider than the seat at the beamiest part. The fore and aft parts tapered sharply. I was tentative for the first mile, then tried some full-pressure strokes. *Oh, yes.* She was fast. And then *Oh, no.*

It always seems to take forever from the moment you know you're capsizing until you're underwater. Then time becomes urgent until you're bobbing beside the boat.

My first thought was to see if I'd broken any part of the fragile shell. No. Having dumped me, she'd righted herself and was floating peacefully with a gallon of water in the cockpit. My second impulse was to look around to see if anyone was watching this embarrassing scene. All clear. Then I tried to remember the remount drill. Getting back into a canoe is comparatively easy—you grab the far gunwale and slither over the near gunwale. Getting back in a single shell is more complicated. There are two nine-foot oars dangling from the oarlocks, so the first step is to gather the handles and put them butt to butt so you can pull on them with one hand. Then you give a huge frog kick and try to launch your body out of the water and up and over the seat. The trick is to turn in midair so your ass lands on the seat. Easier said than done. I was way too tentative the first two tries. Not enough of a kick, not enough of a tug on the butt-to-butt oar handles. I thought for a while, then told myself to stop overthinking. *Just take a breath and go.*

I got into the seat, but I was lying on one hip, one leg splayed out over an outrigger, the other over the side. The oar handles were still in one hand but out of reach of my other hand. I was balancing the boat by wiggling my feet, not sure what to do next. It was at this moment that another sculler came round a bend. He stopped and said cheerfully, "That's one."

"One what?"

"One of the three times you'll tip over. It usually takes

three. But here's the good part—after three you won't worry about tipping over, and you can just row." He added, "If you let go of your death grip on the oar handles, you can sit up and get one in each hand."

That last part was right. As was the part about tipping over three times. I got two and three out of the way before the cold weather set in. Two was when I hit a buoy with an oar blade; three was when a beaver smacked his tail so loud my arms jumped and I caught a crab.

Over the next several seasons I got occasional lessons from three very good scullers. Brett, who coached the novice men's and the women's Virginia eights, was the most poetic. "On the recovery, don't just get your hands away. Imagine you're a heron spreading his wings."

Veronika Platzer, also a coach, was heartily German. She once yelled from her launch, "Stop! Stop! It is too painful for me to watch what you are doing with your hands!" But three sessions with her knocked a minute off my five-kilometer time.

Cécille Tucker, who'd rowed in the U.S. women's quad in the Atlanta Olympics, was very polite at first. We would take out a double, she rowing behind me. "Mr. Casey, engage your lats first." A common failing of male rowers is to yank the oars with the shoulder muscles. This hunching up makes for an uneven drive of the blades. After another mile I did it again. Cécille said, "Oh, for God's sake, John! Remember you've got a neck!"

Rowing—in my single, in a double, in a quad (four scull-ers), in a coxed four (four sweep rowers), and once in a while in an eight—was my main sport in my fifties and sixties. I acquired a steady partner in a double, Tom Allan. He and I raced against each other in two long races. He beat me by a few seconds, then I beat him by a tick. He bought a double for us, which he christened *Passing Wind*. He even bought us two baseball caps with *"Passing Wind"* embroidered on the front. When we traded up for a faster double, he named her, to my relief, *En Passant*. He was even more avid than I. Years before, he'd rowed for Penn and then spent some time with the Olympic squad.

Tom was a bit taller than me and had a more powerful upper body. I could match the length and strength of his stroke because I'm a bit more flexible and have thick quads.

Over the years we raced on lots of lakes and rivers, most frequently on the Potomac and the Schuylkill, sometimes in our age bracket but once in an over-thirty race with no age handicap. We got a bronze medal, as satisfying as our six golds out of eight tries at the Head of the Potomac and the silver at the Head of the Schuylkill. We did better during the fall season of head races, usually about three miles. Brett explained that in a thousand-meter race a single mistake makes a big difference. "And you guys usually make a mistake. In the head races you can make up for a bad stroke."

Twice Tom and I rerigged our double as a pair and raced at the Master's Nationals. The pair has two rowers, each with one twelve-foot sweep oar. Since sweep rowers move in a slight arc, leaning to one side at the catch and pulling through to one side at the finish, the pair requires exact synchrony. The most famous world-class pair rowers are brothers—the Abbagnale brothers. The pair is slower than a double, but when the boat is set and both oars are in sync, rowing her is dreamlike. We won a gold in Topeka, with Tom stroking and me in bow. It's an oddity of the pair that the bow oar has more leverage, so the stronger rower is in the stern. Tom and I went back and forth in an amiable way over who was stronger. On our second try at Oakland, California, Tom was in bow. We were doing okay, holding on to third. I could see five boats behind us. I asked Tom how far out of second we were. It's the bow rower's job to look ahead every so often and act as cox—perhaps call for a power-ten or say it's the last two hundred meters. It's the stroke oar's job to keep his mouth shut and his eyes in the boat. Tom didn't answer right away, so I turned my head. The boat is so precariously balanced that the slightest shift of weight can screw things up. I caught a crab. By the time I dug my oar blade out, we were in sixth place. We got it going again, made a furious sprint. Furiously is not the way to row a pair. We did pass the fifth-place boat, but we weren't going straight and missed the bronze by half a boat length. When we caught our breaths we apologized simultaneously: "I caught a crab." "No, I pulled off course." "I shouldn't have tried to look." "No, I should have steered . . ." Alphonse/Gaston, Gaston/Alphonse.

Tom and I rowed together for nine years without a cross word.

There are many reasons to keep doing sports into middle and even old age—health, vanity, endorphins, adventure—but another good reason is a partner. Tom brought lists of RBEs (really boring exercises). I kept track of our weekly mileage and aerobic points. But when we got in the boat we had confidence that in every training session and in every race each of us was giving maximum effort.

In our eighth head race on the Potomac, with a mile and a half to go, I heard Tom groan. Another stroke and he stopped. He said, "I'm sorry, I'm sorry." And then, tearing the words out of his chest, he said, "I can't."

We learned later that he'd torn a muscle and, even worse, ripped a tendon off his hip bone. At the moment he stopped, I knew it was something drastic. I felt a sympathetic shock—

not sympathetic physical pain but a wordless complete knowledge of what his spirit felt.

I only vaguely remember rowing us to the dock. I don't remember whether I had to help him out of the boat or who helped load the boat for the drive home. We stopped for lunch. He took another couple of ibuprofen pills, all we had on hand as painkillers. It wasn't so much the pain that he minded.

I said, "If we'd hit a log and broken the skeg . . . If we'd broken a rigger . . ."

"It's not the same."

"It is."

"We've never argued."

"Okay. Right. But I know . . ."

"You okay driving the whole way?"

"Yeah."

"Thank you." In the car he said, "I'm going to take a nap. Thank you for trying to cheer me up."

Even after lots of consultations and therapies, Tom wasn't able to row competitively. I'd come to rely on him, as much for his spirit as for boat speed. I went back to sightseeing in my single.

I did train for the head of the Potomac the next year with a very good partner. Halfway into the race a couple out for a holiday in a rental canoe was suddenly alarmed at finding themselves on a racecourse. They panicked and cut across our bow. We collided. Our starboard oars were pinned under their canoe. They sat there, blinking bovinely. I'm afraid I went into Captain Bligh mode. My partner suggested more reasonably and understandably that they put their paddles in the water and take a stroke. We got free, but the dead stop took about twenty seconds. We lost the race by fifteen seconds. I thought the Potomac was putting a jinx on any boat I was in.

It was just as well that I had to go to Rome on translation business. A footnote to the list of reasons to exercise occurs to me. The best cure for jet lag is a four-mile jog. Or even a brisk three-mile walk. It also helps with the fits of melancholy that in my later years have begun to accompany jet lag—or perhaps it's just the sight and sound and smell of a familiar but haunted place. There I was in Rome on a perfect fall day, trundling my bag along a street I knew well—in fact, there was the café I used to take my two younger daughters to—and suddenly I felt my face sag, my chest fill and then empty. *Lacrimae rerum*—the tears of things, or a big boo-hoo about everything. I unpacked in my small bare room at the convent—more economical and quieter than a hotel—and trotted across the Tiber to Trastevere. My legs felt like fifty-five-gallon oil drums. At the end of a side street there was my old gym, still with its wonderfully garbled name in American: Muscle-Body Club. Twenty minutes of exercise there, ten minutes back to the Aventine Hill, a shower, a stroll to the boo-hoo café. But now—how nice it was to be in Rome again.

Stowe, Vermont, 1995

Nell, now grown and living in New York, needed a break. So did I. She'd heard of a hotel and spa in Stowe, Vermont.

Nell swam in the indoor pool and got kelp wraps. I went cross-country skiing, but the snow was slushy, so I hit tennis balls thrown from a machine on the indoor court. Then I saw in a brochure that there was a ski instructor offering telemark lessons on a nearby slope. I showed up with my cross-country skis, thinking that they'd do. No. The instructor rented me a pair of wide downhill skis but with a Kandahar binding. You can run the cable around your bootheel and under a hook and ski using christie turns, as they used to be called. You can also unhook the cables and lift one heel or the other to do telemark turns in a deep genuflection.

The instructor and I went up in a chairlift. He said, "First, let's see how you ski with your heels clamped down—regular parallel turns."

Okay. It came back some. The instructor called to another instructor, "Hey, Joe. Watch this guy." I was puzzled. We got to the bottom. The instructor told Joe to get a video camera. He asked if I'd mind doing another run. He said it wouldn't count as part of the hour's instruction.

He and Joe followed me down, Joe skillfully skiing with the camera, both of them saying encouraging things. I had a flicker of hope that I'd found an unexpected moment of skiing grace.

The instructor said, "Thanks. That was excellent. Now for the telemark."

I had to ask. "When you said 'excellent,' what did you mean?"

"Oh," he said. "We're putting together an archive. We have videos of every style going back to 1954. We were missing the Arlberg technique. That stiff reverse shoulder, the big weight shift. It was like finding a relic."

"Ah."

"So I'm guessing you learned to ski in 1951."

I thought, *Relic.* But why spoil his archaeological fun? I said, "Very close: 1952."

"Well, you made my day."

He must have noticed the shadow that had crossed my face when he said "relic." When I finally did something resembling a telemark turn, he said, "You're catching on. You must have Scandinavian blood."

He was an excellent instructor and basically a good guy—he knew to put a drop of balm on a ruffled minor vanity.

Aerobic Points

Kenneth Cooper's *The Aerobics Program for Total Well-being* was a seminal book in fitness literature. It's clearly written but fairly long. It has a fair number of encouraging sermons, and some anecdotes about dedicated exercisers. I'm going to summarize the core of it in a couple of pages.

1. The standard caution: see your doctor before starting any exercise regimen.
2. For minimum cardiovascular health, get thirty aerobic points per week. For walking a mile in twenty minutes you get one aerobic point. Walking a mile in fifteen minutes gets two points. Jogging or walking a mile in twelve minutes, three points. A ten-minute mile gets four; an eight-minute mile, five points. A six-minute-forty-second mile, six points. A five-minute-thirty-second mile, seven points.
3. If, instead of walking or jogging, you prefer to swim or bicycle, there's an easy way to assign points. Swimming is four times *less* efficient than walking/jogging. So swimming a quarter-mile equals a mile on foot. Bicy-

cling is three times *more* efficient. So you need to go three
miles to get the aerobic points of going a mile on foot.

Yes, some swimming strokes are more efficient than others, but let's not quibble over minor issues. Cooper thinks the
breaststroke should earn only eight-tenths as many points as
the crawl. If you have to swim to shore from a sinking boat,
you might choose the breaststroke to conserve a bit of energy.

And yes, some bicycles are more efficient than others, but if
you're not racing it's not worth the math.

A point Cooper doesn't address is ice-skating or Rollerblading. I figured out from looking at Olympic records that speed
skating is two times as efficient as running. From personal experience I'd guess that Rollerblading is also about twice as efficient.

Cross-country skiing and sculling are about as efficient as
walking/jogging, so a mile is worth a mile. I found that when
I rowed my single shell five miles at a decent clip, it took
forty minutes, about the same as a five-mile jog. Yes, a contrary wind or current makes it harder. I'm obsessive about my
weekly points, but I don't worry about wind or current. Over
time it evens out. Eight-oared shells, fours (four sweep oars),
doubles (two rowers, four oars), and quads (four scullers) are
faster than a single, but I don't do fractions of points. During
the winter on a rowing machine I count 2,000 meters as a mile
rather than 1,600 meters, and this penalty evens out the time
I spend in quads or eights.

In cross-country skiing the quality of the snow makes a difference, as does choosing the right wax, but the disadvantage
of slow snow or less-than-perfect wax will be evened out by
fast snow and good wax.

For tennis, squash, soccer, basketball, and other games,
Cooper is a bit arbitrary. For tennis he gives one and a half

points per set, but of course some sets are longer and/or harder than others. When I play tennis I take my pulse occasionally, and it averages out to very fast walking. It's up after a long rally; it's down after a few short points. For squash my pulse averages about the same as it does when I am jogging.

For circuit training, calisthenics, or weight lifting, I take my pulse and compare it with jogging or walking. If I'm stuck in a hotel without a gym I do a twenty-four-minute routine, alternating push-ups with jumping jacks, pull-ups with doing the Charleston or an Irish jig, and so forth. I give myself the equivalent of a two-mile slow jog. Sawing wood, splitting logs with a maul and wedge, or chopping with an ax is aerobically about the same as a slow jog.

Two subjects Cooper doesn't address: flexibility and strength. My rowing club has an auxiliary yoga instructor during the winter. Good idea. I found that back in my serious tennis-playing days, I played better when I stretched. Light stretches before, long stretches after. As for strength training—recent medical research shows that the old view that you can't build muscle after the age of fifty or sixty is wrong. My sports doc says a lot of over-seventy people can add strength. So tote that barge, lift that bale . . . maybe not endorphins, but *some* kind of a rush. Just be sure to breathe.

•◆•

To recapitulate: the formula for aerobic points is one per mile for walking, two for walking fast, three for a slow jog, four for a jog, five for loping, six for running, and seven for a five-thirty mile.

For swimming, a *quarter*-mile equals a mile on foot.

For bicycling, *three* miles equals a mile on foot.

Thirty aerobic points per week is minimal conditioning for cardiovascular health.

Fifty or seventy-five keeps you ready for vigorous weekend games.

One hundred points means you're in good shape. Ready to climb Mount Katahdin.

More than that is for serious endurance events.

•◆•

If you're training hard, take your pulse first thing in the morning. If there's a rise of more than ten beats per minute (from fifty to sixty-five, for example), you've overtrained. Take it easy for a day.

Along the Way

Running, walking, canoeing, rowing, or standing still, I keep seeing animals. In Pike County, Pennsylvania, there are lots of black bears. I've always liked and admired them, been scared only twice. One time I was fishing for trout in the Sawkill. I'd caught six, needed one more for a supper party that evening. I hooked the seventh, was playing it carefully as it zigged and zagged and jumped. I heard a cough. The largest black bear I'd ever seen was wading into the stream from the other side. Thirty feet away. It had gray hair on its neck and yard-wide chest. Usually if you say a few words in a normal voice a black bear will shy away. Not afraid, just uncomfortable. Yelling at close quarters is likely to rile him. I said, "You are very big." The bear kept coming. The trout made a run toward me, and I raised my arms to keep the line taut. The bear stopped in midstream, looked me over from bottom to top. One of the bits of advice I'd gathered from the guys at the gun-and-tackle store about a close encounter with a bear is to make yourself look bigger. I'd done this by accident. I think the bear had been attracted by the trout's splashing and hadn't connected me to the trout, just thought the trout was in trouble and would be an easy meal. The bear thought for a while, making rumbling noises. I imagined he was thinking that even if I looked eight feet tall, he could still chase me away from the trout. My hands began to shake. I said the first thing that popped into my head: "You've got all the cards."

I felt like an idiot, but the bear turned away. He took a few steps. He stopped and swung his head around for another look at me.

The trout gave up. I stooped to put a thumb in its mouth, my forefinger through the gills.

When I looked up, the bear was gone. Whatever noise he made going through the brush was covered by the stream running over the rocks.

I gathered my rod and basket of fish and walked up the hill to my car. I would have run, but I was completely hollowed out.

•◆•

The other scare was when I was jogging on a dirt road and a cub scrambled out of the woods just ahead of me. It saw me, stood still, and then ran up to me like a puppy wanting to be petted. For an instant I thought, *How cute.* My next and wiser thought was, *Where's the mother?* I hoped she was in the woods ahead of me. I turned tail. The cub playfully followed me. I ran faster. When I looked back after a fifty-yard sprint, the mother was in the middle of the road, ambling after her cub. I was glad to see she was ambling. Black bears, for all their bulk, can easily outrun humans. I didn't stop sprinting until I was well down the road.

There are very few attacks on humans by eastern black bears.

Almost all of them come from a human getting between a sow and her cub. A few come from a male during mating season when the males are in befuddled states of arousal. Another few come when a human is walking a dog. Bears really dislike dogs. They'll go after them as often as they'll run away from them. If Fifi gets scared and runs to jump in her owner's arms, the bear will focus on the dog. Better tell Fifi she's on her own.

That's advice that's hard to take. A bear wandered onto the lawn in front of the family house in Pennsylvania. My mother-in-law's small poodle charged it, yapping. Luckily, the bear was adolescent, probably half-grown, maybe two hundred pounds. The bear climbed a tree. He didn't use the branches, just used his claws on the trunk. In three one-second moves he was thirty feet up. He sat on a branch, hugging the trunk, mewing with fear. I got the poodle inside, but the poor teenage bear didn't come down until after dark. One or two years older, the bear might have knocked the poodle into the next county. Two years younger, the bear's mother might have. Lucky poodle. But the variables are variable. One of the many disservices Disney movies have done is to make wild animals humanoids. They aren't. Even the U.S. Forest Service with its Smokey the Bear mascot is infected. Wild animals are better served by Wittgenstein: "If a lion could talk, we would not understand him."

There are people who are woods-wise who can predict what an animal is likely to do in some situations. Most animals have stances or even facial expressions that can be decoded, but even the canniest and most experienced humans know how ultimately opaque human-animal communication is. Better to wonder, wonder carefully.

One of the most embarrassing and idiotic scenes in *Secre-*

tariat is that of the poor actress who's been directed to look into the horse's eyes and pretend the horse and the woman are reading each other's minds, that the woman is inspiring the horse to win the Belmont. There is, very likely, affection. But a race plan? Even if the woman could whinny, the horse still couldn't understand her.

The trainer, played by John Malkovich, says that he's been training horses for thirty years and he still doesn't know what's going on in their heads. As an actor, Malkovich is in the same league as Christopher Walken for wonderfully unsettling affect, but he delivers that line with straight believability.

What we humans can do is watch. I was putting a canoe in the upper Delaware River when I saw a bald eagle swoop down to catch a fish. Osprey can plunge into the water and swim in it. Eagles can't. They have to lower their talons and pluck the fish out. This eagle went into the water. He or she couldn't get back into the air. The eagle looked around and then headed for the far shore, doing a graceless butterfly stroke, heaving itself along. Halfway there it had to take a rest. I was rooting for the eagle. I even crouched a bit in case the eagle might be embarrassed. Okay, I'm prey to occasional anthropomorphism. The eagle made it to a rock and hopped up. I was surprised to see it still had the fish in one fist. It spread its wings and flapped once or twice, not enough to dry them. It hopped from rock to rock until it was onshore. Out of the blue an all-brown eaglet landed alongside. A juvenile but almost as big as the eagle. The eagle handed over the fish. The eaglet flew off with it, without so much as a thank-you. Okay, I gave in again, but I drew back to reconsider. I have no way of knowing whether the eagle was *choosing* to go to this great length to feed its offspring—what I assumed was its offspring—or whether the effort was instinctive, an automatic program. All I can do is admire the eagle's recovery from the accident, admire the improvised swimming, admire the tenacity, the literal tenacity. The story is clearer without the thought balloons.

·◆·

I've come across snakes fairly often. One time I stepped onto an old wharf on an island off Georgia. The end of the plank I stepped on began to slide. I blinked and saw that it was a snake, a water moccasin. I felt the "zero at the bone." I couldn't move for the whole time the snake poured off the end of the plank, an endless snake, an endless ten seconds.

But another time when I was hiking in the Blue Ridge, I saw a snake rear up a yard in front of me. It wasn't a yard long, and I knew that snakes can strike only about half their length. It was one of the most beautiful colors I've ever seen—an orange copper. I'm pretty sure it had just shed its skin, which is why the color was so vivid. It was, in fact, a copperhead. It was coiled with about eight inches of its length in the air, the head motionless. We looked at each other for a long time. I didn't feel the zero at the bone, just serene admiration. I have no way of knowing whether I conveyed that serenity. Perhaps it was only because I was motionless that after a while the snake uncoiled and slithered very slowly into the brush. I've thought later that it would be good to learn not just to hold my body still but my thoughts as well, to look without a babble of commentary.

Another time I was glad I didn't hold still. I was jogging on a dirt road on the right side. I heard an abrupt crackling whir in the grass. I jumped sideways, all the way to the left side of the road—much farther than I could if just jumping. Rattle, jump. Not a hundredth of a second in between.

A valuable lesson from my short session with Tom "Tracker" Brown was how to get ready to look. Let your eyes unfocus. Unfocused eyes have greater peripheral vision. If something stirs or is a variant color, focus.

I've seen a barely discernible blacksnake inching its way up the dark bark of a locust to crawl into a bird's nest. I've noticed crystallized maple sap where a red squirrel had gnawed through the bark to make a bit of maple syrup. I've caught a glimpse of the shadow of a trout on the pebble bottom of a stream. Hummingbirds hidden among the trumpet vines. I wish I'd learned that unfocus/focus lesson much earlier in life. Now I have to take off my eyeglasses to unfocus, put them back on to focus. As awkward as the eagle doing the butterfly stroke. I'm willing to improvise awkwardly to catch glimpses of animals.

Ben Franklin wanted the wild turkey to be our national bird. I think the wild turkey lost out because it strikes lots of people as comical. As a flier, it's as aerodynamically improbable as a bumblebee. I admire its flying, but the most admirable turkey trait is the male display. I was hiking up a grassy slope when I saw a gaggle of female turkeys. They saw me and fluttered a bit. A tom turkey strode out of the woods on stiff legs. He herded his harem into the woods, then came back out to deal with me. He flared his tail. It wasn't the rainbow display of a peacock, but the blacks and grays were gorgeous. He rattled his fan and pranced in a tight circle with little hard steps. I thought, *I've seen that strut somewhere . . . Yes. Mick Jagger.* The turkey was better at it. Jagger doesn't have the tail feathers. I said, "You are the grandest tiger in the jungle," and he danced again, pivoting and prancing and vibrating his magnificent tail. I made myself smaller and backed away down the hill.

All those creatures and many more. Perhaps the best reason to go for a hike or a jog isn't the aerobic benefit but what you'll see along the way.

Delaware Canoe Trip, First Leg

A river, even a small stream, makes me wonder, Where does it go? Where could it take me? A brother-in-law (we're married to sisters) and I got a map and thought, We could paddle from my cabin on the upper Delaware River 120 miles to Philadelphia, then into Delaware Bay, take a right into the Chesapeake and Delaware Canal, and head south to our father-in-law's farm near Annapolis, Maryland. Could we do about 250 miles in a week? I bent pipe cleaners along the curves of the river and straightened them along the mileage scale. I kept getting different results. Benjamin, twenty years my junior and a triathlete, said, "Let's go to Philadelphia and see."

After finding a good bowman, the next thing is a good canoe. Eighteen feet, Kevlar, only thirty-four pounds. Shakedown cruise of fifteen miles. Eleven minutes a mile. Exuberance.

Noon, day one. The Delaware Water Gap, often visited and painted in the nineteenth century, is still gorgeous, even with an interstate crossing it. The steep, dark hills are so closely set that the perspective is foreshortened as in an old Chinese landscape painting. As soon as we'd got through the water gap, it began to pour. Water came down our sleeves as we lifted our arms to paddle. Water came down our collars. Three inches of water around our feet. Where the hell are we? The map, tucked in my pocket instead of in the waterproof bag, was mush. We hauled the canoe out and drained it. Pulled ourselves up the bank by roots and branches. Found a church-benefit hot-dog sale under a tent. Portland, Pennsylvania. Nowhere near our first-day goal. We shook ourselves dry and devoured hot dogs. Knee-deep in the river to relaunch, I was shivering. We were cheered by a flock—a *swarm*—of swallows swooping and dapping the river.

The rain stopped. Flat water and wooded banks. We paddled farther. Three little boys told us we were in Belvidere, New Jersey. Go on? Too dark. I found the Hotel Belvidere a half-mile up the hill. White Carpenter's Gothic. The hotel owner let us stow the canoe in a storage room. Hot-shower bliss. Pizzeria. Bed bliss.

Breakfast at Uncle Buck's. Stacks of pancakes and sausages. (We ate five thousand calories a day, lost weight.) Old guy at next table said, "I live on a steep hill. Right over Foul Rift. Sit on my front porch and laugh my head off at upside-down canoes. Foul Rift is the first rapids you'll come to. Stick to the Jersey side for the first half, then cut hard for the Pennsylvania side. Some make it."

We hit a set of rapids soon enough. Not so bad. We paddled. Benjamin said, "But I didn't see a steep hill." I said, "These old guys . . ." and stopped. We both said, "Oh, shit."

There was a jagged wall of white water, waves jetting up between boulders. We couldn't see the end. Halfway I yelled to Benjamin, "Pull right! Harder!" We paddled furiously for the Pennsylvania side. "Last bit and we're through!" Except for a ledge between the boulders. We hung, teetered, then swept through on our beam end and rolled over. The current pulled our shoes off. We scissor-kicked the canoe to shore. I cut my foot on a rock.

At noon we got to where we'd hoped to get to the night before.

Easton, Pennsylvania, on one side, Phillipsburg, New Jersey, on the other. Phillipsburg had an easier landing place. I limped up to find a drugstore to get a bandage. Phillipsburg is a sorry town. Abandoned factories, stores closing, Social Security office open.

But the sun was out, and we were drying in the breeze. We slowed only when we saw a bridge. A bridge meant a narrow place, and a narrow place meant white water. Benjamin, way forward in the sharp bow, felt as exposed as a ball-turret gunner. At the sight of a bridge he would start to dab rather than stroke. I'd crane to see which line to take.

Still not many towns, only every seven miles or so, but we were getting into the boutique zone—teatime meal was bruschetta and smoked salmon. Heading for New Hope, Pennsylvania, but where were we? Climbed up to find a road sign. Centerville. Only four miles from New Hope, but it was getting dark. There were some quaint inns, all closed for the season. We stashed the canoe in the woods, thought of walking to New Hope. Because Benjamin's good-looking, and because I was limping, a woman gave us a ride. Next morning for the same reasons we got a lift back to the canoe. Flat water to New Hope. Met a woman in a single scull. She said, "Watch out for the dam. There's a chute on the left. Kayakers do it for thrills." We'd had enough thrills. Benjamin reconnoitered, found a canal that took us around the dam and the boulder field below it.

Lunch at Washington's Crossing. Warning: dangerous rapids at Trenton.

We lost an hour while Benjamin scouted on foot. Hard to get passersby to talk—we looked battered and feral. We pushed on. Nothing but a few jounces, then tidewater.

Trenton is only twenty-five miles from the north edge of Philadelphia, but for a lot of those miles there is almost nothing but woods. A factory or two. A yacht club. Mostly the big wide river and woodland. Around a bend we see a mountain of coal and there's the black stern of a freighter, the *Clipper Stamford* out of Hong Kong. In case she backs up, we zig to the other bank. Out of nowhere—three shots. No whine of bullets. Shotgun? Overhead a vee of geese, heading south. A wingbeat or two later one plummets into the water. Amazing splash. We zag back toward the Pennsylvania side.

The sky is turning violet. Benjamin has to get back to work the next day. We're sure we're almost to Philadelphia, but we have to find a suburb, a town—someplace where Benjamin's wife (who is conveniently visiting their daughter in Haverford, Pennsylvania) can pick us up. We pull harder, gurgle along. We've reached that tiredness in which the body is moving of its own accord. It's the red-shoes effect—can't stop dancing.

A beautiful seawall on the Pennsylvania side. An acre of perfect lawn. A mansion. In the dusk we make out a man pushing a lawn mower. He stops, starts to roll it toward a shed. Benjamin sprints. I hold the painter and melt into the seawall. The river, now running out with the tide, is lovely as it darkens. I don't want to leave it.

Benjamin comes back and says, "Guess whose house this is." I have a crazy hope that it's someone one of us knows, who'll give us a beer, a sandwich.

Benjamin says, "William Penn."

That's even better. This could be the very seawall where the Lenni-Lenape brought their pelts after canoeing down from pre-Milford. The groundskeeper is just closing the gate to the estate, now a museum. He thinks we're twelve miles from Philadelphia by car. He's never been by boat.

I say, "Close enough."

Benjamin says, "Annapolis next spring."

Seventieth Birthday

After the first three-day leg of the canoe homage-to-parents-in-law trip, I let the end of October and all of November go by in mild jogging and sawing and splitting wood. I was busy preparing for the spring term and re-re-rewriting a novel. It came as a surprise that my seventieth birthday was coming up. I said that I didn't want a party, that I wanted to spend the day in solitude. I wasn't being grumpy or melancholy. I'd hiked fifty kilometers at age fifty (bless the metric system). A seventy-kilometer hike seemed likely to be monotonous. Bless the mechanical advantages of wheels and blades. Five weeks might be enough time to train. I started bicycling to the gym, rowed on the ergometer, Rollerbladed. Bicycling (as noted earlier) is three times more efficient than going on foot. The rowing machine is one for one. Roller-blading I figured was about twice as efficient as jogging, as is ice-skating. I compared the records of speed skaters against runners—the ratio checked out, more or less, and if hockey skates aren't as efficient as speed skates, so what? I did a bit of everything except ice-skating, but I did do the math and figured out the distance around our local ice-skating rink.

On my birthday I bicycled to the gym. I forgot my pass—biked back for it. Did twelve and a half kilometers on the erg, got impatient and pushed a bit harder than planned. Biked home for a snack of peanuts and blueberry juice, biked to ice rink. It was crowded—I forgot it was Saturday. Easy pace. Bright spot was when a woman linked her arm in mine and said, "You must be from up north." I skated with her for a bit, mentioned my seventieth-birthday plan. She lost interest.

I finished those leisurely five miles and turned in my rental skates. As I unlocked my bicycle, a beggar asked for spare change. I gave him my old Windbreaker. My wife showed up with my Rollerblades. She said, "You gave him *that*? After you'd been sweating in it . . ." I said, "I had on two layers underneath it." But she had a point. The beggar was using it to sit on. I bicycled to the 2.2-mile paved part of the Rivanna Trail. I was going to do six lengths, 13.2 miles or—I should have brought along pencil and paper—call it 21 kilometers. It was the happiest event of the day. No one out for a walk. I was swooping along, my hands laced behind my back, just the whir of the in-line wheels, the Rivanna murmuring on one side, tree leaves on the other. I came around a curve and saw a walker headed toward me. I glided so as not to take up the whole width of the pavement. It was my ex-wife. She called out, "Happy birthday!" Amused and cheerful.

A mile later I ran into a pile of twigs and leaves, clogged up the skate wheels. Cleaned them with a twig and swooped on. I felt mentally tired only when I turned around after 4.4 miles and set off to do the same route again and again. A few strides and the rhythm and the cold air moved me into the pleasurable part of the red-shoes effect—legs and body angle automatic, eyes unfocused but alert (a Tom "Tracker" Brown helpful hint), and mind as content as if waking up in bed from a good dream. The second and third circuits were a breeze, but my fingers were clumsy unlocking my bicycle. Only about four miles to go, but I'd forgotten that they were mostly uphill. Dusk gave way to dark. I put on an orange reflective vest. I allowed myself the lowest gear. Stop signs and red lights broke the rhythm. The last hill felt so steep it made me laugh. I leaned my bike on the front porch railing and went into the dining room. On an index card I jotted down miles and translated into kilometers. Recalculated. The total kept changing. To be on the safe side I picked the number that fell short by . . . five kilometers? I got back on my bike and coasted to the Charlottesville High School track. Went around and around, keeping track by starting in lane six and moving in a lane every lap. Back uphill. More math. Okay—3.5 miles, about 5.5 kilometers. Still short? I walked the dog around a one-mile block. For some reason I took my cell phone. It rang. It was my eldest daughter calling to wish me a happy birthday. After a minute of conversation she said, "Dad? Are you drunk?"

"No. I'm walking Eloise. Last mile. Just to make sure. I'm having trouble with the math."

"Oh, okay. Your birthday kilometers. Are you all right?"

I sang, "'We are marching to Pretoria . . .'"

She said, "Call me as soon as you get home."

After supper I recalculated using an actual calculator. It turned out I hadn't needed the extra bicycling. It came out to seventy-five kilometers and change. I decided not to count walking the dog, since we'd stopped a lot for her to sniff the neighborhood dog news.

The event hadn't been all that arduous. I wasn't stiff the next day, not nearly as much as after the marathon or the fifty-mile hike run or even the fifty kilometer, or a twenty-kilometer rowing race in an eight. My giddiness when I was walking the dog was possibly as much due to low blood sugar as endorphins. There was some exhilaration at having taken a measure of myself, however moderate. It did turn out to be a building block for three more events over the next year.

Delaware Canoe Trip, Second Leg

A year later I cartopped the canoe to Trenton. Benjamin and I spent the night there in a motel and hired a cab to drive us to Pennsbury Manor at four a.m. The driver, an Afghani, was pleased to hear we were canoeing from our mother-in-law's house to our father-in-law's. He approved of family ties and pilgrimages. It also seemed to give him confidence in the way we lashed the canoe on top of his cab.

We put in at four-thirty a.m., top of the tide. An easy distance for the first day. Pleasant paddling past small towns and yacht basins. The tallest buildings in Philadelphia came into view, and we thought we'd be there in an hour. After an hour, the buildings didn't seem any closer. It began to get hot. The buildings disappeared. We came round a bend, and we were abruptly on the Philadelphia waterfront. I spotted a motel where I'd stayed when racing on the Schuylkill. We pulled into a yacht basin. The guy in charge wanted us to pay as if our eighteen-foot canoe were a yacht. Next marina the same. The third place we put in was flanked by two abandoned warehouses and, on the street side only a hundred yards from the motel, an office building. There was a ramp leading to the street. When we were halfway up the ramp, a man warned us off. He disappeared. Benjamin, a law abider, suggested we move on. We did. The next marina also had an office building along the street. I persuaded Benjamin to carry our knapsacks while I put the canoe on my neck and shoulders. I said, "We can go through the double doors."

I got into an empty office. A man came in. He was startled to find an eighteen-foot canoe going by his desk. Then he laughed and said, "Let me hold the door for you." He walked us through the building and onto the sidewalk.

The desk clerk at the motel asked us for our license-plate number. We pointed to the canoe just outside the glass doors. She shrugged and said, "It won't fit in your room." We carried it to the parking lot, where the attendant, who had a West African accent, was as interested as the Afghani cabdriver in our trip. He patted the canoe and said we should store it next to his shed. "No one will touch it, I promise you. I like what you are doing."

The next morning, at four-thirty a.m., there was a fine rain. No one up and about, so we carried the canoe down the forbidden ramp. *Ha!* When we got on the river, the wind picked up. We put in once again at the top of the tide, but it hadn't begun to run hard. It was eerie—lots of lights in the city, but the river was dark. My theory was that we'd get a bit more current in midstream than at the side.

Near Camden, New Jersey, the light from the oil refineries' vent flames and beacons was swirled in the wind-driven rain. The Delaware Water Gap had been a beautiful Chinese landscape, but this was more beautiful—as beautiful as the wildest Turner painting. I was so mesmerized, and at such length that Benjamin turned around and said, "John, I beseech you. Get us out of the shipping channel."

Indeed. We couldn't see far enough ahead to avoid a ship or its four- or five-foot wake. We got close enough to the Port of Philadelphia piers to look up at the names of berthed ships. *Aegean Glory, Maersk Harmony.*

Then came sheets of rain. We had to pull onto an islet to dump the ankle-high water. The river was turning into a wide bay, and we weren't sure which way to go in the next-to-no-visibility. We heard a roar. We finally recognized the sound—a jet plane landing at the Philadelphia International Airport, a third of the way to Wilmington. The invisible jets served as an audible aid to navigation.

By the time the airport was off our stern, Benjamin was proved right—there were ships coming upstream. A friend of mine who'd been a lighthouse keeper a bit south of where we now were had written me, "Delaware Bay is simultaneously the most boring and the most dangerous body of water on the Atlantic Coast of the U.S." Among the dangers he mentioned were the shoals that were just far enough below the surface to be invisible but near enough to make waves break or create unpredictable eddies.

The closest we came to capsizing was when we turned into the sizable wake of a ship, aiming to take it at a slight angle, not head-on. The wake came toward us; we paddled toward it. We didn't see the underwater shoal. We reached it just as the wake broke over it. The canoe rode up nicely into the boil but came down hard into the trough. We'd learned after Foul Rift to use our paddle blades as outriggers, which kept us upright for the sled ride. We paddled hard to get past the shoal and onto the next wave before it broke. Another abrupt up and down, some pitching and rolling, but we were clear.

A thing I knew but hadn't thought of: islets and points of land don't end at the waterline. The islet is just the above-water part of a below-water ridge. So we steered clear of visible islets, but how to avoid the completely invisible shoals? One answer is that there aren't shoals in the shipping channel. A correct but dangerous answer. Next answer: hug the shore—but not too tightly, since the shore is the biggest shoal of all. But at least we could get safely to land, even if upside down.

Just before the sun burned off the mist, a long, sleek kayak came across our bow. It was the only craft our size we'd seen since New Hope. The kayaker was headed for shore, intently windmilling his genuine Inuit paddle.

No more ships in sight. We stopped for a lunch at a desolate industrial site. Some off-color liquid was draining into the mud. We ate in the canoe. Then we had a taste of the boring part, paddling parallel to I-495. We were now hours out of Philadelphia, and the tide was going to turn. We put on some speed to get to the Port of Wilmington. We reached the mouth of the Christina River at slack water. Benjamin had two questions: (1) How far to Wilmington? (2) Where could we stash the canoe for the night? Answers: (1) Farther than we thought. (2) The Lord will provide. We paddled past a lot of ships and cranes, then past some woodland. There was a confluence, and luckily we chose to go left. We saw a small boathouse and a man putting in a single shell. I said, "Let's ask."

I said to the man, "How do you like your Hudson?"

He looked up. "Fine." He looked at my Rivanna Rowing Club tank top. "What do you row?"

"A Van Dusen."

We did some more back-and-forth, mentioned some names. In the small rowing world there are far fewer than six degrees of separation.

We came to the crucial question: Could we stow our canoe in this boathouse? He said, "I'm afraid not. I'm locking it up for the season. But if you follow me, I'm going up to the Wilmington Rowing Club boathouse. That'll work out. I'm the coach."

Another slow mile or two and there was a huge boathouse. After we put the canoe inside, the man asked what time we'd be leaving. Five a.m. was perfect; he was taking out an eight then. He said if we'd follow him upstream another three miles, he had a spare bed and a couch at his house. We thanked him, but another three miles up and then back in the morning . . . He gave us a tip on a cheap motel only a mile away on foot, and on a good place to eat.

We strolled along the riverfront, working the kinks out. Benjamin said, "It is as if you're both Freemasons."

A hot shower, another stroll to crab cakes and beer. To bed at twilight.

•◆•

The coach and a crowd of rowers wished us good luck. The trip back down the Christina River was the best part of the third day. After that it was hot and unchanging all the way to Delaware City. A long lunch to wait for the tide to go our way again through a small barge canal that linked to the Chesapeake and Delaware Canal. When we got to the big canal we didn't have more than fifteen miles to go, but the temperature rose to ninety degrees, and the headwind felt hot and stuffy. The canal is straight and unrelenting. The tugs pushing barges put up only moderate wakes, but the powerboats—motor yachts ranging from thirty to fifty feet—churned out steep high waves. The drivers often didn't know the rules of the road and would cut across to take a look at us. Some of the time there were stands of old pilings nearby, and we'd race to get behind them. We used up a lot of energy and time running away from the wakes of motor yachts. And where the hell was Chesapeake City? We got more and more tired. There was no red-shoes effect, just doggedness. We got there but not with enough steam to be pleased that we'd reached the state of Maryland. Benjamin had to get back to work, so he got a local taxi to take him to the Wilmington train station, a short trip along the hypotenuse of the triangle of which we'd paddled the two legs. I had a room in a quaint bed-and-breakfast. I arranged for someone to drive me and the canoe to Trenton to retrieve my car and take the canoe back to Milford, Pennsylvania. After supper I sank into bed, stunned with sun and fatigue. The next day I was back in Milford in five hours, including loading, unloading, and reloading the canoe. It seemed a mockery.

But the day after *that,* as I waded into the Delaware River to launch my single for a short row, I stood for a while in the current. I was still a little drunk or hungover from paddling in rain and sun. I dipped my hand in the water. I knew where it was going. Our trip was an homage to our parents-in-law, but also, it occurred to me, to the river. Before it was renamed the Delaware it had many names in Algonquin. My favorite is Lenapewhihituck—the Swiftwaters of the Lenape.

One Thing Leads to Another

Irowed my single on the Lenapewhihituck/Delaware River another ten times, not sure why, just that it was a pleasure to do six miles faster than I could in a canoe. It was in multiples of 1.5 miles, the rock-free bit of river above and below Milford Beach. Nine minutes downstream, thirteen minutes up, the swift waters of the Lenape. After each leg, spin the boat and do it again.

When I got back to Charlottesville I ran into my old rowing coach and pal Brett, now running a locally grown produce business. He asked if I was fit. He hadn't rowed for a few years, wanted some variety from his four-mile morning runs plus all-day hikes on weekends. He also wanted an adventure. He suggested we do the Wye Island race (12.5 miles) in a double. If we averaged our ages, seventy and forty-four, we'd be well into the masters' over-fifty category. We started training. The Rivanna Club doubles weren't always available, members before guests. I was still a member, but Brett wasn't. He'd founded the Rivanna Rowing Club twenty years earlier when he was the Virginia women's and novice coach. He thought, with some justification, that it would be a nice gesture for the club to make him an honorary member. No dice. I'd have to pay a guest fee each time we trained. I did this a number of times, but it was getting expensive. There was a high-school boathouse on a smaller reservoir nearby. Their coach offered us a double that we could use in the evening after the high-school practice was over.

I wouldn't have missed the Beaver Creek Reservoir for the world. Brett and I would get there at dusk and row the 1,100 meters eight or ten times. Very hard. The only rest was when we'd spin the boat. One night there was a mist on the water, only a handful of stars visible straight overhead. Either by keeping count of the strokes or by instinct, Brett knew when to stop before we ran out of water. Rowing in a bowl of mist was eerily beautiful. The boat *felt* fast. I thought that the mist streaming around us might just be giving us the illusion of speed, but when we checked our watches it turned out that even with the turnarounds we'd done almost seven miles (okay, 6.875 miles) in forty-five minutes. Heartening.

On non-Brett days I rowed my single nine or ten miles, steady state, lower rating. Good for getting used to long distance.

The Rivanna Rowing Club had a rule that any boat entering the Wye Island event had to do a practice 12.5-mile race. It was scheduled six days before the Wye Island Regatta. Brett and I thought it was a bit too close to the event, but we ponied up Brett's guest fee and squared off against the Rivanna mixed eight. In theory an eight, even a mixed eight, should leave a double well behind. Brett and I weren't angry about the stringent bookkeeping, but it was just enough of an irritation to be helpful. After a fast start, we settled in to a good rhythm. The air was cool and still, the water smooth. We got into that state of grace rowers call *swing.* At the catch I heard all four oar blades drop into the water with a single note—a short liquid chink—then the rising note off the stern as the wake gurgled faster during the drive. The three of us were in tune, Brett, I, and the boat. Sometimes it can be like that.

The Virginia men's coach was on the dock when we pulled in after finishing. He looked up the course. He said, "So. Where is the other boat?" We didn't say a word.

Race day was windy. Even off the water among the cars and vans and boat trailers, there were unpleasant gusts.

The Wye Island Regatta is open to boats of all kinds— not just racing shells but fixed-seat rowboats as well as a fleet of kayaks and canoes. There were even a couple of dragon boats. The boats started in their different categories at ten- to twenty-second intervals. The singles went off before us, so for the first mile we threaded our way through them. We were the first double. The other doubles hung with us.

I'd pinned a map of the course to the back of my tank top so Brett could navigate, but I'd screwed up the readout from the impeller. It showed strokes per minute and boat speed but not kilometers traveled. Brett knew where we were for the first four miles by landmarks—a bridge, a pier, a headland with a house—but when we came to more open water it was hard to tell. We'd left some doubles behind, but one was tailing us. The wind picked up and made enough of a chop to cut the boat speed. The gusts also kept fluttering the map so that Brett found it hard to read. What he *could* do was give a few gruff barks during the bouncy part. "Drive through it!" "Lengthen!" And his old coaching favorite: "Row like you mean it!" And then, "Oh, *yeah*! All the way home, just like this!"

Somewhere past the chop we took a ten-second break to gulp Brett-ade—water and honey with a pinch of salt. We barely lost boat speed. Not a clue where we were, but the boat felt light and swift, and *that* was the point.

"Home stretch. Let's build over four on this one. That's one . . ."

Later Brett admitted he'd been guessing. It wasn't the last mile, more like the last two miles, but he was right to call for more speed. His enthusiasm was as much a boost as overtaking another boat would have been.

A hard turn to port around a long point, a straight line to another point jutting into the channel, hard turn to starboard, and Brett sings out, "I see the finish line! Let's go!"

I saw later on the nautical chart that that last straightaway is 1,500 meters. Brett said, "Oh, yeah!" several times, a better spur than a spur.

A blast from a Freon horn signaled that we'd crossed the line. The rule was to row sixty more strokes past the finish in case there was another boat coming. Nothing in sight. We glided a hundred yards, not able to move. I have no memory of how we got from the finish to the launch site. There's no dock. You embark and disembark in thigh-high water. Someone held the boat. Brett's hands were bleeding. I couldn't move my legs over the gunwale to get out. I used my hands to lift one leg and then the other, and then had to hold on to the boat to stand up. After a bit we were able to lift the boat and put it on a rack. With very small steps we went up the slope, picked up the pace when we saw a table of sandwiches and fruit juice. "Oh, yeah." Drank, ate, stretched. I massaged my quads. Brett went to find something antiseptic and anesthetic for his hands.

When the results were posted we weren't surprised to see we'd won the over-fifty category. We were surprised to find we'd beaten the over-forty, the over-thirty, and a lightweight college double. To put this in perspective, the Wye Island race, while it attracts lots of rowers, is too close to the prestigious three-mile head races (Potomac, Schuylkill, Charles) to be a sensible preparation for the college crews and rowing clubs looking for major competition. It takes too long to recover. It would be like a miler running a marathon a week or two before his prime event.

The week after Wye Island it felt good not to do anything— just walking the dogs and sawing firewood. I got restless again. I did some moderate rows in my single, but I missed someone pushing me hard; Brett had been a strong tonic. When some of the Rivanna rowers suggested I join them for coached sessions in the erg room at the boathouse, it seemed a whimsical oddity—twenty people on rowing machines going nowhere while watching their readouts on a tiny screen.

I thought back to twenty years earlier. When I was fifty-one I'd done a killer eight-week erg training program set up by Brett. Six days a week, two of them two-a-days. Each week the three hard days got harder and the long days longer. I remembered Wednesdays—pyramid day. Warm up for two thousand meters. Then do one minute to get up to speed, four minutes at cruising speed, three minutes at head-race speed, two minutes at short-race speed, one minute at top speed. And then go back down the pyramid, two minutes, three minutes, four minutes. What was hardest wasn't the one minute of going all out, or even the two-minute. It was the second three minutes of head-race speed. Over the eight weeks Wednesdays got harder, first by adding a two-thousand-meter steady-state piece after the pyramid. The next week another pyramid—and so on, until by the next-to-last week, there were three (three!) pyramids with a four-minute rest in between. The Thursday prescription was "Do something fun for an hour," but it had a footnote: "Keep heart rate at one-twenty." The next-to-last Friday was twelve one-minute intervals at race pace. (Earlier

Fridays were five five-minute pieces, four four-minute pieces, and so on. The twelve one-minute intervals were the hardest. It was usually the ninth one that made me reconsider the whole enterprise.)

I forgot Monday. Four seven-minute pieces, each Monday a bit faster. The sixth Monday I didn't think I could face doing it alone on my old erg in the dark basement. I went to a small gym. It was primarily a women's gym with a large studio for aerobics, but there was an up-to-date ergometer. I asked one of the two women trainers to come by during the third seven-minute piece, the one during which there seemed to be no end in sight. I said, "If you could just do a little cheerleading for a minute, it'd help."

The first trainer got into it in a sweet way: "Come on! Come on! You can do it! Only another two minutes! You can do it, you rowing god!" The other trainer laughed. I would have laughed, too, except my quads were hurting.

The other trainer, a Valkyrie, thought this looked like fun. She came over during the last seven-minute piece. She knew something about ergs. "What's that I see? You're pulling one-forty-nine? Don't give me that crap! I want to see one-forty-eight, you piece of scum!" And then the old favorite, now on T-shirts, at that time a novelty: "Pain is weakness leaving the body."

And then she called for one-forty-seven, one-forty-six.

"It's willpower. Use your damn *will*!"

Done. She reached past me and pressed "Memory" on the computer readout. "There. Good boy. Negative splits." Negative splits are when each five hundred meters is faster than the one before. She said, "So who's more fun—Terry or me? You better say me."

I went back the next Monday, but the Valkyrie had moved

on. The sweet cheerleader tried to be a Valkyrie, but she was an aerobics instructor at heart. "Whoo! Looking good!" At the end of the eight weeks I went to an erg competition and won in the over-fifty category. The prize was an Everlast vinyl gym bag. During the drive home I coughed up something dark. The erg in my basement gathered dust.

All that was twenty years earlier. Now I was seventy-one. Why on earth would I do it again? Nothing to see along the way but tiny numbers. No herons or kingfishers.

The two coaches made it worthwhile. Even experienced rowers have bad habits. They can have little hitches in technique that need to be noticed by someone who knows how to fix them. Or they can get mental blocks—*if I'm going this fast, I must be hurting, I must be hitting a wall* . . . A really good coach can intuit when a rower is hearing an inner voice that foresees failure prematurely.

Both weight-lifting coaches and track coaches agree that to get better you have to surprise your body. Years before I'd read about an East German coach who'd trained a Russian sprinter. The Russian had reached a plateau. No matter how many one-hundred-meter sprints he ran or how many times he ran the same set of stairs in a stadium, he didn't get faster. The East German told him to run odd distances. Sometimes the coach didn't tell him how far the distance would be—just start him with a whistle and stop him with a whistle. The Russian won the bronze in the hundred meters at the Montreal Olympics in 1976.

We'd warm up for ten minutes on our ergs, then do abdominals of seven or eight different kinds—crunches, bicycle abs, trunk-rotation abs, more abs . . . Another warm-up, and then the surprises. Sets of 1,000 meters. Sets of 333 meters at race pace with twenty-second rests, then with fifteen-second rests.

The guy on the erg next to me did the math—333 meters is one-sixth of the 2,000-meter standard erg race. By the time each session was over we'd done more than 12,000 meters at every speed from cruise to all out. Cool down and stretch.

One evening the surprise was a relay race. Two teams of eight, three rowers jumping on ergs to do 1,000 meters, then jumping off to jump on the next erg when someone finished. The strategy was complicated, but the idea was to have the stronger rowers row more pieces than the slower ones. What was impressive was that the coach picked the teams so carefully that at the end of about twenty-five minutes, the difference was only four seconds.

The sessions were on Tuesdays and Thursdays, but if you wanted to improve—the coaches kept track and were enthusiastic about better times—you had to put in two or three aerobic days and another day of shorter and faster pieces, either on an erg or running hills.

The guy on the erg next to mine asked me how old I was. He said, "Good. We need someone in the over-seventy race." He added, "I'm fifty-five, but my biological age is twenty-nine." After that he started glancing over at my readout during a piece or two. "Come on, John. Hang with me on this one." He rubbed some club members the wrong way, but he struck me as being an interesting variety of jovial.

Sometimes the physical side peps up the mental. Once in a while it's the other way around. The days before the competition, I was in a good mood. I'd finished—at last!—a long, long project. The students in my classes for the spring term were smart and fired up. I drove to Alexandria, spent the night in a bargain-price motel. It was snowing in the morning. The radio news predicted a record snowfall. Let it snow, let it snow, let it snow. The T. C. Williams High School gym was filled with ergs—a hundred or more. In front of each bank of ten there was a large screen—about the size of a screen in an art-movie theater. Each of the ergs not only had its own tiny read-out but was wired to a cartoon boat on the big screen, so all the rowers could see where they were in the pack. I watched for a bit, thought the big screen was a funny and ingenious carnival touch. I went to the warm-up room, ran into guys I'd seen over the past twenty years at regattas, ran into boys wearing the colors of my old high school.

I said, "I went there."

One of them said, "When?"

"I graduated in 1957."

One of them said, "Before I was born."

The math whiz among them said, "Before my *parents* were born."

I thought that was yet another variety of jovial. I was in an unsquelchable good mood. Warmed up slowly, did a few fast bits, cooled down.

I got in my erg in the row of the really old guys, seven or eight of us, as compared to the hundreds in the young categories. I looked up at the big screen. There was my little #3 boat. I got suddenly jittery with nerves, had dry mouth. Years earlier a Virginia coach had told me that pre-race nerves are useful. They pump adrenaline through you. You should burn it fast; it lasts for only twenty strokes. Use it to get off ahead, then settle into your race plan.

I did get a jump. There was the little #3 boat inching her way across the big screen, nothing but white ahead of her. I felt lighthearted approaching the 1,000-meter mark. I remembered the worst thing a coxswain had said to an eight I'd been in. "We're halfway . . ." *Okay, take a big ten and don't look at the damn halfway mark. And four more before taking a peek. Good.*

Nobody making a move. Keep it long. Take it up a notch before *the 1,500-meter mark. Oh, yeah. And take it up again. Burn it all.*

A curious thing is that your quads hurt less, everything hurts less, if you're passing another boat or, as in this case, you're leaving another boat behind, even a cartoon boat on a screen. Maybe the elation brings up another drop of adrenaline—use it. You can go rubbery and wobbly afterward.

Done. I kept rowing very lightly to get rid of lactic acid, but soon there were more rowers waiting to take our seats. I walked around the gym. I thought of a story a colleague had told me. A friend of his, another writer, spent some time in a fishing village in the Dominican Republic. He ordered a rowing machine from the United States. When the truck dropped it off, it was enough of an event that his neighbors gathered. "What is in the box, señor? A rowing machine? How wonderful! Could we get one such as yours to put in our boat?"

The writer spoke fluent Spanish, but it took him a very long time to explain.

I thought of Iowa farmers who'd been irritated at Plimpton and me for jogging four miles around the section. I thought of the words of a hymn: "Come, labor on! / Who dares stand idle on the harvest plain, / While all around him waves the golden grain?"

Long drive home on uncleared roads. The next day I shoveled snow. A Charlottesville city ordinance requires home owners to clear the sidewalks in front of their property. I did mine and a neighbor's. I cleared the fifty-yard dead-end side street so that my other neighbors could get out. "Come, labor on! / Who dares stand idle . . . ?" A friend called to ask if I would help her dig out her Volkswagen. It was buried not just by fallen snow but by the waves of snow the city plow had flung up. We groused about the damn foolishness of that, then found it laughable, then found a companionable pleasure in excavating the VW, carefully prying plaques of crust off the windows as though uncovering a relic. By the time we were done the sun was shining on the foolery, and the last strains of that damn puritanical hymn were gone.

I went cross-country skiing. Not good snow, but the late-afternoon winter light was still and clear. Heading home in my tracks I got going just hard enough so that my breath made ice in my beard.

From my seventieth-birthday seventy-kilometer event through the three-day canoe paddling, the Wye Island race, and the ergometer sessions and the Mid-Atlantic Erg Sprints, and several days of shoveling, it had been a lot of one thing leading to another. It was time for a diminuendo.

I got a phone call that evening. An official of the Mid-Atlantic Erg Sprints told me that my time in my age group qualified me to go to the C.R.A.S.H.-B. erg championships. The C.R.A.S.H.-B. event is a big deal in the open category— rowers from all over the world. Even in the older categories it's a national championship. The official offered me a round-trip plane ticket to Boston and a hotel room. There was a temptation. An athletic scholarship! At my age! I could ask Brett to devise another killer training schedule—eight workouts a week, two-a-day on Tuesdays and Fridays.

"I'll call you back."

What decided it for me wasn't the thought of the physical effort—it was the time it would take in mental focusing. I thought about it a lot, but it would come just at the time the spring-semester teaching always becomes intense. I also had a story to rewrite. After my first shot at a rewrite, all I could do was scrawl at the bottom of the last page, "Make it shorter and funnier." An unhelpful comment, no matter who made it. Getting it right would take some musing, not speed work.

I went back and forth about the C.R.A.S.H.-B.'s. Out of the blue I remembered—saw and heard very clearly—Cyril Ritchard as Captain Hook in a 1960 television version of *Peter Pan*. On the quarterdeck of his pirate ship, elegant in frock coat and three-cornered hat, he looked into the far distance and crooned, "Ah, fame! Thou glittering bauble . . ."

Why this wisp? If it was a message, it was pretty oblique. Try this reading: Hey, you're a middle-of-the-pack guy. You're lucky to have had a good year; you're lucky to be still at it. Medals? Medals are for wind chimes. What you love is the grace of rowing or paddling or skiing, to connect with the grace inherent in boats or skis, and the grace with which they move on water or snow. You do the indoor-gym stuff to stay ready. Sure, exercise gets blood to your brain, but it's the time outdoors that alerts your senses.

I said, "Thank you. It's a great offer. It's just that the timing isn't right."

As I think back to that decision, I wonder which of the reasons to exercise that offer left out. Health? Vanity? Endorphins? They were all there. Competition? That was certainly there. Getting out in the elements? Not at all. But another factor was missing. It's a factor I didn't realize plays an important part in the list of good reasons to exercise. All the exhortations to exercise start with the standard warning "Consult your doctor" and end with the advice, "You won't stick with it unless you find a sport or exercise you really like doing." Okay, I know that. But as I remembered mentors and companions from Monsieur Rupik to my canoeing partner Benjamin Warnke, I saw how lucky I've been to find someone who said, "Here's something we could do. Are you ready? Are you game?" What I didn't fully know is that it is not important just to find something you like doing but also to find someone with whom you like doing it.

One of the reasons I'm not going to celebrate birthdays anymore—or, for that matter, New Year's—is that I see people talking themselves into getting old. It's not quite as much a folly as trying to remain forever young—e.g., imagining oneself still able to play contact sports or be able to do the *prisyadka,* that Russian squat-and-kick dance. I'm trying to stay somewhere between buying into the predeterminations of the calendar and the folly of denying aging altogether.

I do wonder what would happen if I gave up those energy-burst races. Would I have to give up catharsis, that purification through total effort? Or would I redistribute catharses among the other intensities of life? Spend more time "along the way" and less doing "intervals"? Can't tell yet. All the reasons to exercise physically still apply—health, vanity, endorphins, adventure—but some of the other reasons are shining more brightly. There are the utilitarian: digging garden beds or sawing and splitting wood, the "Come labor on" Puritan satisfactions. There are also the playful, which could be tango lessons or playing tag with grandchildren. "Buffalo gal, won't you come out tonight . . . and dance by the light of the moon."

And there are the companionable. Soon Benjamin will be calling about the last leg of our canoe trip.

Acknowledgments

Thanks to my editor, Carol Janeway, and my agent, Michael Carlisle, both of whom urged me on at just the right moments. Scott Aronin, Henry David Thoreau, Monsieur Rupik, Hal Greer, David Plimpton, Jed Williamson, the H-20 Slocum Watch, Marcel Proust, Bonkers & Alice, John Irving, Johnny Caldwell, Roger and Marie Chapman, Lenny Chesney, Bill Keough, Jane Barnes, John Rowlett, Hurricane Island winter course, Harold Varmus, Connie Casey, Tom "Tracker" Brown, Captain William Tongue, Leigh Hancock, Hannah Holtzman, Liz Lee, Kurt Vonnegut, Kevin Sauer, Brett Wilson, Veronika Platzer, Cecille Tucker, Tom Allan, Tom Jones, Maud and Nell Casey, Kenneth Cooper, Jeffrey the poodle, Rosamond Casey, and Benjamin Warnke.

A NOTE ON THE TYPE

The text of this book was set in Garamond No. 3. It is not a true copy of any of the designs of Claude Garamond (ca. 1480–1561), but an adaptation of his types, which set the European standard for two centuries. This particular version is based on an adaptation by Morris Fuller Benton.

TYPESET BY

Scribe Inc., Philadelphia, Pennsylvania

PRINTED AND BOUND BY

R. R. Donnelley, Harrisonburg, Virginia

DESIGNED BY

Iris Weinstein